W0246570

Establishing Private Health Care Facilities in Developing Countries

WBI DEVELOPMENT STUDIES

Establishing Private Health Care Facilities in Developing Countries

a guide for medical entrepreneurs

Seung-Hee Nah and Egbe Osifo-Dawodu, MD

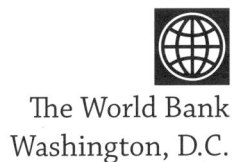

The World Bank
Washington, D.C.

© 2007 The International Bank for Reconstruction and Development/The World Bank
1818 H Street, NW
Washington, DC 20433
Telephone: 202-473-1000
Internet: www.worldbank.org
E-mail: feedback@worldbank.org

All rights reserved
First printing June 2007

1 2 3 4 10 09 08 07

This volume is a product of the staff of the International Bank for Reconstruction and Development/The World Bank. The findings, interpretations, and conclusions expressed in this paper do not necessarily reflect the views of the Executive Directors of The World Bank or the governments they represent.

The World Bank does not guarantee the accuracy of the data included in this work. The boundaries, colors, denominations, and other information shown on any map in this work do not imply any judgement on the part of The World Bank concerning the legal status of any territory or the endorsement or acceptance of such boundaries.

Rights and Permissions
The material in this publication is copyrighted. Copying and/or transmitting portions or all of this work without permission may be a violation of applicable law. The International Bank for Reconstruction and Development/The World Bank encourages dissemination of its work and will normally grant permission to reproduce portions of the work promptly.

For permission to photocopy or reprint any part of this work, please send a request with complete information to the Copyright Clearance Center Inc., 222 Rosewood Drive, Danvers, MA 01923, USA; telephone: 978-750-8400; fax: 978-750-4470; Internet: www.copyright.com.

All other queries on rights and licenses, including subsidiary rights, should be addressed to the Office of the Publisher, The World Bank, 1818 H Street, NW, Washington, DC 20433, USA; fax: 202-522-2422; e-mail: pubrights@worldbank.org.

Library of Congress Cataloging-in-Publication Data

Nah, Seung-Hee
 Establishing private health care facilities in developing countries : a guide for medical entrepreneurs / Seung-Hee Nah, Dr. Egbe Osifo-Dawodu.
  p. cm.
ISBN-13: 978-0-8213-6947-0
ISBN-10: 0-8213-6947-4
ISBN-10: 0-8213-6948-2 (electronic)
 1. Health facilities--Developing countries--Planning. 2. Health facilities--Developing countries--Design and construction. I. Osifo-Dawodu, Egbe, 1965- II. Title.
 RA395.D44N34 2007
 362.109172'4--dc22

                          2006103080

Cover and publication design: James E. Quigley, World Bank Institute.
Cover photos: Alan Gignoux (Lebanese hospital); Yosef Hadar (Brazilian researcher); John Isaac (Indian surgeon); Eric Miller (Mozambique doctor and mother); and Dr. Jean-Marcel Guillon (Franco-Vietnamese Hospital, Ho Chi Minh City).

Contents

Foreword ix

Acknowledgments. xi

Abbreviations. xiii

Chapter 1: Introduction. 1

   So You Want to Build a Hospital?. 1
   Recent Trends in Health Care 3
   Overview of Health Care Facilities 6

Chapter 2: Project Concept and Mission Statement 13

   The Whats and Whys of Your Project. 13
   Project Concept 13
   Mission Statement. 15
   Project Management. 16

Chapter 3: The Prefeasibility Analysis 19

   Better to Stop Now than Fail Later. 19
   Conducting the Prefeasibility Analysis. 20
   Key Questions 20
   Risk Assessment and Management. 25

Chapter 4: The Feasibility Analysis 29

   Finding and Clearing a Path to Success 29
   Conducting the Feasibility Analysis 30
   Nonfinancial Analysis 31
   Financial Analysis: No Margin, No Mission. 52
   Will Your Hospital Be Viable?. 65
   A Note on the Business Plan 66

Chapter 5: Obtaining Financing **67**

Keeping Your Fuel Tank Filled 67
Keys to Success in Obtaining Financing 68
How to Look for Financing 70
Types of Financing 73
Structure of Financing 76

Chapter 6: Marketing Your Facility **83**

If You Build It, Make Sure They Come 83
Developing and Refining Your Marketing Strategy 84
Building and Maintaining the Hospital's Reputation 91

Chapter 7: Facility Planning and Design **95**

Time to Start Drawings 95
The Facility Design and Planning Team 96
Space and Functional Programming 102
Conceptual (Preliminary) Design 103
Schematic Design 103
Consider Future Expansion 105
Cost Projections 105

Chapter 8: Major Medical Equipment **107**

Not Everyone Needs an MRI 107
A Systematic Approach 108
Selection Criteria 108
Procurement 116
Delivery and Installation 120
Training 121
Maintenance and Insurance 122

Chapter 9: Facility Construction **123**

As Planned, on Time, and on Budget 123
Planning for Construction 123
Construction Assignment 129
Construction Documentation and Construction Contract 130
Insurance Requirements 132
Time to Break Ground 133

Chapter 10: Facility Opening **135**

Preparing for the Big Day 135
Staffing 136
Documentation of Operating Policies and Procedures 137
Building Commissioning 138
Medical Equipment 139
IT System 139
Operating Licenses and Permits 140
Minor Equipment and Supplies 140
Insurance 141

The "Hotel Management" 142
Training and Support System for Troubleshooting 143
Dry Runs. 143
Opening Day Preparations 144

Appendix A: Sample Timeline for Building a Health Care Facility. 147

Appendix B: Millennium Development Goals. 151

Appendix C: Types of Public–Private Partnerships 153

Appendix D: Health Status Indicators 155

Appendix E: Health Facility and Hospital Development. 157

Appendix F: Evaluating and Selecting Hospital Consultants. 163

Appendix G: Typical Provider Payment Mechanisms 169

Appendix H: Different Forms of Business Ownership 171

Appendix I: Sample Project Cost Estimation Summary 175

**Appendix J: Summary of Project Costs and Financing Plan for a
Greenfield Hospital Project. 177**

Appendix K: Sample Format for a Financial Projection Model 179

Appendix L: Sample Outline for a Business Plan 191

Appendix M: Selected Examples of Financing Sources 201

Appendix N: Additional Information on Preferred Shares. 203

Appendix O: Programming Individual Departments or Services. 205

**Appendix P: Criteria for Selection of Medical Equipment
and Products. 211**

**Appendix Q: Sample Table for Construction Cost Estimates
by Category 215**

Appendix R: International Competitive Bidding. 221

**Appendix S: Parsons META Hospital and Health Care
Construction Pitfalls 223**

Appendix T: Sample Job Description for Director of Nursing 225

Appendix U: 10 Rules for Planning a Hospital. 227

Suggested Reading 229

Tables

1.1. Private Health Expenditure as a Share of Total Health
Expenditure, 2002 5
1.2. Overview of Facility Types 8

Boxes

1.1. São Luiz Hospital and Maternity, Brazil 3
1.2. Prime Cure Group, South Africa 10
1.3. Asian Eye Institute, the Philippines 11
1.4. Fleury Diagnostic Center, Brazil................................. 11
2.1. Excerpts from Sample Mission Statements 16
3.1. Challenges of Catchment and Competition 25
3.2. Protecting Your Business through Insurance 27
4.1. Accreditation of Health Care Organizations: JCAHO and JCI 40
4.2. The Importance of Design Functionality.......................... 47
4.3. Physician Shortage Limits Services............................... 50
5.1. Dealing with Foreign Exchange Risk............................. 75
6.1. Unique Characteristics of the Health Care Market................. 86
6.2. A Marketing Innovation: Franco-Vietnamese Hospital's
Medical Card.. 89
6.3. Targeted Marketing Efforts: The Apollo Hospitals Group 92
8.1. ECRI: Advisory Services on Health Care Technology................ 113
8.2. Leasing Medical Equipment: One Hospital's Experience 117
8.3. Faulty Packaging Delays Delivery 121
9.1. Parsons META: Advisory Services on Development of Health
Care Facilities 126
9.2. Saving on Costs through Construction Management 127
10.1. Pareto Analysis and Inventory Management 141
10.2. 10 Common Mistakes to Anticipate and Avoid 144
10.3. A Success Story: The Opening of Reddington Hospital 145

Figures

Project Management: Establishing a Private Health
Care Facility... 17
Step-by-Step Approach to Planning, Procurement, and
Management of Medical Equipment 109

Foreword

There is growing awareness of the role of the private health sector in many low- and middle-income countries. Countries in these income brackets represent 84 percent of the world's population and 93 percent of the disease burden, and 50 percent of health expenditure in these countries is private. As a result, many governments are rethinking the role of the private sector, including both the commercial and not-for-profit subsectors, in enhancing the provision of high-quality and efficient health care. High-performing systems tend to feature mixed delivery of services, with private providers playing an integral role. An appropriate regulatory framework and strong government participation in health care financing are essential in enabling the private sector to make this contribution.

The environment for development of private health care facilities is becoming more favorable in other ways as well. In the context of rapidly growing economies, health insurance schemes or other risk-pooling mechanisms are increasingly common. Some developing countries such as Thailand, India, and South Africa have identified the health sector as a strategic sector for international trade. They are developing "health tourism" centers that are becoming competitive with similar facilities in high-income countries.

Many physicians and other health care providers dream of establishing a private health care facility, seeing it as the culmination of their professional success. Unfortunately, many such dreams have not been realized—often because the entrepreneurs were not familiar with all that would be required to build and operate such a facility. In particular, many medical entrepreneurs lack adequate knowledge about how to source financing from potential investors.

A major barrier to the development of the private health sector is the scarcity of long-term capital. Long-term financing is essential to enable the development of sustainable private facilities capable of providing high-quality care to meet the continuing needs of the population. In many countries, commercial banks view the private health sector as highly risky, and they often are unwilling to consider proposals even when they have sufficient liquidity. The international donor community, until fairly recently, did not engage directly in the private sector, believing these entities could raise sufficient funds on their own.

Drawing on resources from across the World Bank Group and elsewhere, this book aims to provide medical entrepreneurs with some of the tools they need to build sustainable health care facilities for their communities. It offers practical "how to" guidance on key issues such as the project concept, prefeasibility and feasibility analyses, regulatory and policy environment, investment and financing needs, marketing and pricing principles, facility construction, staffing, and risk management. Aimed principally at the new private entrepreneur, the book may also be useful to managers of public or not-for-profit health care facilities who are also grappling with issues of quality, efficiency, and sustainability in health care.

FRANNIE LÉAUTIER
Vice President
World Bank Institute

Acknowledgments

It takes a village to raise a child, and something similar can be said about this book. The authors benefited from the wisdom, efforts, and goodwill of many people, including the many health care entrepreneurs who inspired us to tackle this project. We would like to thank all those who encouraged, challenged, and helped us as we went through this learning experience.

This book would not have been possible were it not for the enthusiasm and persistence of the core members of the team from across the World Bank Group. Isabel Rocha Pimenta made substantial contributions to drafting chapter 2 and selected boxes, as well as to early versions of chapters 6 and 7. She helped to identify external advisers and engage other team members, leveraging her strong organizational skills despite an extremely busy schedule. Ilyse Zable also contributed significantly by participating in early discussions on the book's structure, helping to draft chapters 3 and 4, and reviewing initial drafts of the first four chapters.

We would like to thank Nneka Mobisson, who listened patiently to our ideas in the early days, carried out effective research, and contributed to pulling together the first drafts of several chapters. Her infectious enthusiasm is much appreciated. Rocky Lee was also a great addition to the team, making substantial contributions to several chapters in earlier drafts of the book and drafting chapters 6 and 7. He also created graphic process summaries that helped the team clarify complex relationships between various components of the process for establishing a health care facility. Bob Adeghe brought his real-life experience to bear on some of these issues and contributed to drafting chapter 8 and selected boxes.

Pallavi Kapnadak helped pull the document together, cleaning up the appendixes, assisting with research, and communicating with external parties to obtain permission to use their information. Raj Raina helped prepare the document for editing and did research for the reading list. Kemi Osinusi and Eva Ross contributed at different times to moving this project forward, and Mouna Lahlou, Gbemi Adeniran, and Fatma Rashid helped with administrative tasks. Our thanks to all.

A number of industry leaders and entrepreneurs graciously took time out of their busy schedules to speak or meet with us and to review drafts of selected chapters. In particular, we would like to express our heartfelt gratitude to Dr. Joel Nobel, founder and president emeritus of ECRI, who saw the value of our efforts immediately, during our very first call to him; to Douglas Heisler, founder of the former META Associates and currently vice president of Parsons META; and to Daniel John Olphie III, formerly principal at META Associates and currently vice president of Parsons META. All were generous and open in sharing their vast knowledge and experience with us, and Mr. Olphie also contributed material to an early draft of chapter 7. We are also grateful to Andre Staffa, CEO of Hospital e Maternidade São Luiz in Itaim, São Paulo, Brazil, and Dr. Jean-Marcel Guillon, chairman of Franco-Vietnamese Hospital in Ho Chi Minh City, Vietnam, who shared their experiences, reviewed early versions of selected chapters, and offered invaluable advice.

We thank Frannie Léautier, vice president, World Bank Institute; Jacques Baudouy, former director, Health, Nutrition, and Population, World Bank; Ruben Lamdany, former director, Sector and Thematic Group, World Bank Institute; Bruno Laporte, manager, Human Development Group, World Bank Institute; Guy Ellena, director, Health and Education Department, International Finance Corporation; and Maria da Graça Domingues, director, Department of Special Operations, International Finance Corporation.

For providing written contributions and suggestions, we are grateful to Dr. Kola Olofinboba of McKinsey & Company; Drs. Enoma Alade, Segun Dawodu, Ronke Dosunmu, and Kwesi Boateng, medical entrepreneurs; Dr. Richard Ajayi of Bridge Clinic, Lagos, Nigeria; Jim Rice of the Governance Institute; Cheryl Shapiro, an attorney; and our colleagues at the World Bank Group—Merunisha Ahmid, Imoni Akpofure, Andrew Alli, Ifeoma Ezeokafor, April Harding, Chris MacCahan, Tonia Marek, Emmett Moriaty, Shilpa Patel, Alex Preker, and Karim Suratgar.

Our thanks also go to John Didier, Dana Lane, Ludi Joseph, and James Quigley for their support through the publication and dissemination process, and to Catherine Sunshine for her excellent editorial help.

Lastly, we would like to thank our families for their patience through this long journey.

Abbreviations

A&E	accident and emergency
ALOS	average length of stay
ARV	annual requirement value
CDC	Centers for Disease Control
CEO	chief executive officer
CFO	chief financial officer
CIF	cost, insurance, and freight
CPU	cost per use
CSSR	central sterile supply room
CT	computed tomography
DCO	director of clinical operations
DHR	director of human resources management
DON	director of nursing
DRG	diagnosis-related group
FOB	freight-on-board
FTE	full-time equivalent
HMSL	Hospital e Maternidade, São Luiz
HVAC	heating, ventilation, and air conditioning
IBRD	International Bank for Reconstruction and Development
IDA	International Development Association
IRR	internal rate of return
ISO	International Organization for Standardization
IT	information technology
IV	intravenous
JCAHO	Joint Commission on Accreditation of Health Care Organizations
JCI	Joint Commission International

LIBOR	London Interbank Offered Rate
LLC	limited liability company
MIS/HIS	management information system/hospital information system
MRI	magnetic resonance imaging
NGO	nongovernmental organization
OT	operating theater
PACS	picture archiving and communicating system
PAHO	Pan American Health Organization
RFP	request for proposal
TA	technical assistance
UNICEF	United Nations Children's Fund
USAID	United States Agency for International Development
WHO	World Health Organization

Note: All dollar amounts are U.S. dollars.

1

Introduction

So You Want to Build a Hospital?

This book is a practical guide for medical professionals who are interested in establishing health care facilities in developing countries. It is intended for individuals and organizations with little or no business experience who are seeking guidance on how to turn a general idea into concrete reality. Our goals in writing the book were modest. The guide does not provide an exact roadmap for building a hospital or other type of health care facility, nor is there any guarantee that the new entrepreneur who follows the approach described will be able to obtain financing from investors. Rather, the book is designed as an introductory resource with which to begin the process.

Successful physicians, perhaps in the diaspora, in government service, or elsewhere, may see a need to provide private health care services to a selected population.[1] These physicians, who may be renowned in their fields, often have had limited business experience. In several cities in the developing world there are unfinished and abandoned hospital shells, remnants of the dreams of aspiring medical entrepreneurs. In others, failed hospital projects have gone bankrupt in their early stages after being launched with much optimism.

Establishing a new hospital in a developing country is an extremely risky venture. Experience suggests that it can take from one to three years to prog-

---

1. The "diaspora" of qualified medical professionals who have emigrated from developing countries is very large. For example, between 1986 and 1995, 61 percent of doctors who graduated from one medical school in Ghana left the country. Of these, about 6 percent migrated to another African country (South Africa), but the great majority went to the United Kingdom (55 percent) or the United States (35 percent). D. Dovlo and F. Nyonator, "Migration of Graduates of the University of Ghana Medical School: A Preliminary Rapid Appraisal," *Human Resources for Health* 3, no. 1 (1999): 45.

ress from the initial concept to completion of the feasibility analysis, making it difficult for any entrepreneur to sustain significant momentum during these critical early stages. On average, the time required for the entire project, from definition of the concept to opening of the completed facility, is between three and five years (see appendix A for a sample timeline). In addition, a new hospital typically takes about five years after starting its operations to become fully established and start generating positive cash flows sufficient to service debt and pay dividends.

The information provided here relates to the planning and establishment of self-sustaining health care facilities, whether for-profit or nonprofit (the latter includes nongovernmental, independent parastatal, faith-based, and nondenominational institutions). We want to emphasize the term "self-sustaining," because many facilities are built without due consideration at the outset of their long-term viability in technical, social, operational, and financial terms. Such facilities often fail to live up to their original expectations and fall short of achieving their overall mission and goals, despite being founded on good intentions and sound concepts.

We have chosen to focus on the process of building a hospital, starting with the entrepreneur's idea and ending with the opening of the facility to the public. Building a new health care facility is far more than just a construction or real estate development project, as first-time entrepreneurs inevitably come to appreciate. Our goal is to help reduce both the time spent on this learning process and the number of avoidable mistakes that are made.

In order to illustrate the guidelines in this book, we framed the discussion using as a reference point a medium-size (about 100 beds) secondary or tertiary care hospital that is privately owned and managed on a for-profit basis. Box 1.1 describes one example of such a hospital, which has evolved over a long period of time to become a successful network of hospitals. We have chosen to focus on the medium-size hospital because this seems to be the most common type of facility for which medical entrepreneurs from developing countries seek financing. Clearly, however, given the epidemiological changes and advancements in medical practice described below, entrepreneurs may wish to consider other types of facilities as well.

While we have chosen the medium-size hospital as our model facility type, much of the information can be applied to any health care facility. The health care sector is, however, affected by its local environment, and the guidelines in this book may not apply directly to every context. It is imperative that medical entrepreneurs develop a solid understanding of the local health care environment in which they wish to operate in order to customize the guidelines to apply to a particular situation.

Our challenge in writing this guidebook was twofold. First, we wanted to educate the first-time entrepreneur on the conceptual elements involved in any

---

Box 1.1 São Luiz Hospital and Maternity, Brazil

Hospital e Maternidade São Luiz in Itaim, São Paulo, Brazil is a medium-size hospital and the flagship unit of the HMSL Group. The Group has its roots in a small clinic established by three local physicians in 1938. It currently operates two hospitals in São Paulo, a city of 18 million people. The hospitals provide general medical care as well as specialized care, including maternity and neonatal care.

The Itaim hospital, with 2,800 employees, currently performs about 2,300 surgical operations, delivers about 700 babies, and provides emergency treatment to about 25,000 patients every month. Typical occupancy rates range from 82 percent in the hospital to 90 percent in the maternity clinic. Most patients are privately insured or belong to a health care management organization. The Itaim unit has annual revenues of about $120 million and has received certificates of quality from the International Organization for Standardization (ISO) and the Organização Nacional de Acreditação, the principal health care accreditation institution in Brazil.

The HMSL Group is an example of a business that began as a small clinic run by a few medical doctors and grew to become a leading private health care provider in its country, with good prospects for further growth. It accomplished this by providing patient-oriented, high-quality services, guided by a forward-looking management philosophy. Over the past two decades, the Group has opened its ownership to the physician community in Brazil in order to expand its capital base. Thus a large number of physicians who practice at HMSL hospitals are also equity investors in the Group, although majority ownership is still in the hands of descendants of two of the three physicians who created the original clinic. The Group has also set a good example for hospital management by actively recruiting nonphysician professional managers, implementing quality and cost control mechanisms, and providing training oriented to patient satisfaction. Several years ago, for example, the Group adopted a sophisticated financial management approach that enabled it to take advantage of low-cost, foreign currency–denominated, long-term financing. This also served to shield the business from being negatively affected by the sudden devaluation of the Brazilian *real*.

---

health care facility building project. Second, we sought to explain some of the practical realities and complexities that are commonly encountered during such a project. Appendixes to the book contain samples of the data that need to be collected and analyzed, and a list of suggested readings provides a starting point for more detailed research into specific areas of health care facility building projects.

Please note that the terms "your project," "your hospital," and "your facility" are used interchangeably in this book, as are the terms "you," "project developer," and "project sponsor."

Recent Trends in Health Care

The dynamics of health care demand and supply in developing countries in recent years have led to a growing need for private health care facilities. As a result of various demographic and epidemiological changes, the public sector has been overwhelmed by the demand for health care services, particularly services delivered by hospitals. This has forced changes in government policies that in turn have led to significant increases in private sector participation in health care provision.

Demographic and Epidemiological Changes

Low- and middle-income countries represent 84 percent of the world's population and 93 percent of the disease burden, but only 18 percent of global health spending. Despite significant improvements in general health indicators, vastly advanced medical technologies, and increasing expenditures on health, serious challenges remain in the quest for universal and high-quality health care. Improvement in health indicators appears to have slowed in the 1990s, and at the present pace most regions will not meet the health-related Millennium Development Goals by 2015 (appendix B).

Increasing life expectancy and slowing population growth in many countries are bringing a greater burden of chronic and degenerative diseases such as cardiovascular diseases and cancer. Along with other noncommunicable conditions such as road crash injuries, these diseases of aging account for a rising share of health care demand. They often require comprehensive health interventions. Thus the graying of the population has increased the demand for hospital care in terms of the volume of admissions, average length of stay, and complexity of treatments.

There has been a significant decrease in the share of communicable diseases. However, changes in mortality and morbidity are distributed unevenly throughout low- and middle-income countries. Although the means to control common communicable diseases are available and infection rates of tuberculosis, malaria, cholera, and measles have declined, these diseases remain a major burden to the poorest countries—many in Africa—and to rural and poor populations in several middle-income countries. Special emphasis needs to be placed on the emergence of the HIV/AIDS epidemic, which has brought increased pressure on often fragile health systems. In some high-prevalence environments, more than half of hospital admissions are related to HIV/AIDS.[2]

The overlap of the epidemiological transition and the emergence of new threats such as HIV/AIDS exacerbates the pressures on national health systems at a time when public resources in many countries are increasingly stretched. Given the multiple demands on limited public funds, in several countries it ap-

---

2.   In Swaziland, for instance, 60 percent of hospital admissions are due to HIV/AIDS-related illnesses. U.S. Agency for International Development, Bureau for Global Health, *HIV/AIDS Country Profile: Swaziland* (Washington, DC: USAID, 2004), http://www.synergyaids.com/Summaries_PDF/SwazilandprofileFeb2004FINAL.pdf.

pears that reliance on the public sector alone to address health challenges may not be a viable or sustainable option in the long term.

Expanding Role of the Private Sector

Given the capacity constraints of the public sector in meeting health care demand, many governments are beginning to turn to the private sector and to reliance on market instruments to enhance the efficiency and quality of health care provision.[3] One of the earliest areas of private sector participation (in the public sector) was the subcontracting of auxiliary services such as laundry and cleaning. This was followed by subcontracting of more clinically oriented services and departments, such as radiology and pharmacy.[4]

More recently, health care reforms in various countries have sought to increase the role of the private sector as the provider (although not necessarily the financier) of comprehensive care, to complement the activities of the public sector. The general argument is that these reforms can retain equity in the financing of health care yet promote efficiency by introducing and encouraging competition. High-performing health systems are typically characterized by mixed delivery of services, with private providers playing an integral role. Appendix C briefly describes some different types of public-private partnerships.

Table 1.1. Private Health Expenditure as a Share of Total Health Expenditure, 2002

Region	Percentage of total
Low-income	72.2
Middle-income	50.6
Lower-middle-income	54.6
Upper-middle-income	42.4
Low- and middle-income	53.8
East Asia and Pacific	62.2
Europe and Central Asia	34.4
Latin America and Caribbean	52.2
Middle East and North Africa	42.9
South Asia	76.0
Sub-Saharan Africa	59.5
High-income	36.7

Source: World Bank, *World Development Indicators 2005* (Washington, DC: World Bank, 2005).

3. Until the twentieth century, most people paid independent health providers directly for their services. Thus, in most countries, private provision predates the development of publicly funded health care services.
4. International Finance Corporation, *Investing in Private Health Care: Strategic Directions for IFC* (Washington, DC: IFC, 2003).

Today, the private sector increasingly serves as a partner with public health systems, particularly in the provision of clinical health care. In many low-income countries over 50 percent of health care provision and financing is now private (table 1.1). The increase in private sector participation in health care services, especially in developing countries where public sector capacity is constrained, makes this guidebook a timely resource.

Overview of Health Care Facilities

Health care facilities encompass a wide range of institutions including, among others, general and specialist hospitals, ambulatory care centers, diagnostic clinics, nursing homes, maternity homes, and hospices. The range of delivery models and facility types is greatly influenced by factors specific to country and location, and although facilities can be grouped into different categories, these groupings are not as discrete as they might appear. There is likely to be significant variability within these groupings both by region and by country. As you think about what kind of facility you want to build, it is important to understand how facility types can vary in their resource requirements and in their ability to fulfill operational goals and needs.

Each country has health care delivery models that, while based on international standards, vary according to local considerations such as history, cost, geography, infrastructure, labor market, and provider training. Thus, the specific services offered by different facilities (for example, outpatient or inpatient care) and by different providers (for example, specialists, general practitioners, or nurses) often differ from country to country.

The role of the independent medical practitioner has been the cornerstone of most Western medical systems. In contrast, hospitals have played a much larger role in providing both inpatient and outpatient care in a number of other countries, particularly those that had socialist or communist governments during the second half of the twentieth century. In much of Africa, modern health systems have been based on acute care hospitals, with primary care only becoming widespread since the 1980s.[5]

Advancements in medical technology and practice as well as changes in provider incentives, introduced in many industrial countries as part of their health reform efforts, have resulted in a shift from costly inpatient to more cost-efficient outpatient models of care. This can be seen as many hospitals reduce available beds, merge, or simply close down. For example, according to the American Hospital Association, the total number of hospitals in the United States decreased from 5,800 to about 5,000 between 1980 and 1997. Concurrent with

---

5. World Bank, *World Development Report 2004: Making Services Work for Poor People* (Washington, DC: World Bank, 2003).

this decrease in hospital bed capacity, there has been a trend toward decreasing the length of stay, with a rising volume of ambulatory care and day cases. In the United Kingdom, for example, the percentage of admissions treated as day cases increased from 17 to 35 percent from 1985 to 1996.[6]

In developing countries, the availability of beds varies widely, but in general the shift to outpatient models of care is not quite as marked as in the developed world. Countries that are experiencing an increasing share of noncommunicable diseases as they advance in the epidemiological transition have had to expand inpatient care, especially if they do not have a history of predominantly hospital-based care. This shift is also rooted in the aging of developing-world populations. For instance, in Brazil, the share of the population that is over 65 (about 6 percent in 2005) is projected to double to over 12 percent by 2030.[7] Hospital admissions are likely to rise in tandem with the increased demand for care for the elderly.

A common and useful way to think about health care facilities is to group them in three general categories: inpatient, outpatient, and diagnostic. Table 1.2 provides a brief overview of these different facility types. In practice, facilities exist along a continuum and the differences between the various types are not as sharp as these descriptions imply, but the distinctions have been exaggerated to ensure clarity.

Inpatient Facilities

Inpatient care facilities in many countries can be divided into two broad groups: acute care facilities (hospitals) and long-term care facilities (rehabilitation centers and nursing homes).

ACUTE CARE

Acute care facilities can be subdivided into secondary and tertiary care facilities, according to the breadth and depth of services they provide. Given their provision of the most specialized medical care to the most severely ill patients, tertiary facilities are generally teaching and research hospitals, almost always located in large urban centers. Thus, tertiary care facilities tend to be significantly more complex and costly undertakings to both build and operate than secondary care facilities. The reference facility for this book (the medium-size hospital) belongs to the secondary care category.

6. U.K. Department of Health, NHS Annual Report 1995/1996 (London: Crown Copyright, 1996).
7. United Nations, Department of Economic and Social Affairs, Population Division, *World Population Prospects: The 2004 Revision* (New York: United Nations Secretariat, 2005).

Table 1.2. Overview of Facility Types

	Inpatient care			Outpatient care		
	Acute					
	Tertiary	Secondary	Long-term	Primary/general	Specialized	Diagnostic
Service focus	Single or multispecialty, including highly specialized care (e.g., cardiology, pediatric cardiothoracic surgery)	Single specialty (e.g., maternity) to general hospital (e.g., internal medicine, pediatrics, ob/gyn, general surgery)	Part-time or full-time support services (e.g., living, rehabilitation)	General consultative care	Varies from single specialty (e.g., ophthalmology, gastroenterology) to multispecialty (e.g., comprehensive women's health)	Range of tests to aid in medical diagnoses
Procedures	Complex surgeries with specialized equipment	Simple surgeries (e.g., appendix removal, Caesarean section)	Basic fitness and nutrition (e.g., physical therapy)	Broad preventive activities	Basic treatments and simple surgeries	Noninvasive and simple invasive procedures
Equipment	Sophisticated in-house diagnostic equipment (e.g., MRI, CT scan)	Basic in-house diagnostic equipment (e.g., x-ray, biochemistry)	Basic medical and living equipment (e.g., IV, oxygen tanks, special furniture)	Basic medical and diagnostic equipment	Basic and specialized medical and diagnostic equipment	Mix of imaging and laboratory diagnostic equipment
Typical number of beds	150–500	30–150	30–250	0–20	0–10	n.a.

n.a. = not available

Source: Adapted from *Investing in Private Health Care in India: Funding Robust Business Models*. Chennai, India: Infrastructure Development Finance Company, 2002.

LONG-TERM CARE

Facilities providing long-term care can be subdivided into rehabilitation centers and nursing homes. Rehabilitation centers provide patients with full-time attention as part of lengthy rehabilitation programs following injury or illness; patients are expected to recover and eventually to return home. Nursing homes or skilled nursing facilities usually offer permanent, 24-hour care for patients who can no longer live on their own, although some operate as day care centers for patients who go home to their families at night. In nursing homes, trained professionals provide medical services to residents while other staff assist residents with daily activities such as bathing, eating, and housekeeping. Nursing facilities may specialize in short-term or acute nursing care, intermediate care, or long-term skilled nursing care. As the share of the population that is elderly continues to increase in many developing countries, the demand for all types of long-term care facilities is likely to increase.

Outpatient Facilities

Outpatient facilities can be divided into two main groups: primary/general care facilities and specialized care facilities. The latter provide services that in the past were often provided in hospitals, and the trend toward specialized outpatient care has contributed to the reduction of hospital beds in a number of industrial countries. In certain countries, there exist outpatient facilities that offer both types of services, for example, Prime Cure facilities in South Africa (box 1.2).

PRIMARY/GENERAL CARE

Primary/general care facilities provide primary health care services to a mainly outpatient population. In many developing countries, these facilities tend to focus on consultative services for basic health care. Many public systems have used similar facilities to expand access to allopathic health care in a relatively cost-efficient manner, although with varying degrees of success. For example, in the United Kingdom primary health care centers and "general practices" deliver much basic health care. Because of the low investment required, many solo practitioners (often general practitioners) in developing countries have sought to start such primary facilities, either to provide better care or to supplement their public sector wage, or both. In some developing countries, standardized outpatient care is provided by a network of facilities, usually staffed by general practitioners and nonmedical health staff.

Box 1.2   Prime Cure Group, South Africa

Prime Cure is a multidisciplinary health care organization in South Africa. It has a staff of more than 800 people, complemented by a national network of approximately 2,000 general practitioners and 800 associated health care professionals. It provides services to almost 1 million patients every year, drawn from a broad socioeconomic spectrum.

The Prime Cure group has 45 walk-in medical centers that offer a range of services such as general medical and dental care, optometry, radiology, pathology, and HIV/AIDS treatment. All the doctors, dentists, and other health care providers working at these medical centers are monitored by a peer review system that has been put in place to monitor the treatment of patients, thus ensuring a consistent standard of care. The providers follow treatment protocols and guidelines that are endorsed by experts in the field. Medication for acute and chronic conditions is provided according to a specific formulary. A pathology laboratory provides in-house pathology services to the medical centers and network doctors in fields such as hematology, biochemistry and endocrinology, microbiology, serology, cytology, and histology.

For more information: Prime Cure Group, http://www.primecure.co.za/.

SPECIALIZED CARE

With the shift from inpatient to outpatient care in some industrial countries has come a near-revolution in the delivery of care through outpatient (ambulatory) facilities. In the United States, there has been a significant increase in stand-alone ambulatory care centers, a trend fuelled to a large extent by changes in provider reimbursement as well as by patient preference. These centers include freestanding urgent care centers, basically acute general-practice facilities that provide internal medicine and pediatric services; single-specialty centers such as those in ophthalmology or gastroenterology; and multispecialty centers, such as comprehensive women's centers. Multispecialty centers typically include three to four 72-hour beds, thus blurring the distinction with inpatient facilities. Some developing countries have also started to develop specialized outpatient facilities; one example is the Asian Eye Institute in the Philippines (box 1.3).

Diagnostic Centers

Diagnostic centers are facilities offering services for medical diagnosis, such as specialized imaging (for example, magnetic resonance imaging) or laboratory tests. These may be stand-alone facilities such as the Fleury Diagnostic Center in Brazil (box 1.4), or they may be integrated with clinical facilities. In some hospitals diagnostic services such as imaging or laboratory services are provided by independent entities. Diagnostic centers have seen noticeable growth in many countries in recent decades. In Indonesia, which has many islands, attempts have

---

Box 1.3 Asian Eye Institute, the Philippines

Oscar Lopez, chairman and chief executive officer of the Lopez Group of Companies, recognized the need to bring world-class eye care to the Philippines. His collaboration with Filipino American ophthalmologist Dr. Felipe Tolentino led to the establishment of a state-of-the-art eye care center in the Philippines. Opened in 2001 in Manila, the Asian Eye Institute is the first comprehensive ambulatory center in the country to offer a complete range of services for diagnosis and management of eye diseases, including glaucoma, retina and vitreous diseases, pediatric eye diseases, and adult strabismus, among others. It offers immunology and uveitis services, cornea and refractive surgery, ophthalmic plastic surgery, low vision and visual rehabilitation, and anesthesia. In addition to providing these clinical services, the institute aims to be a specialized training and research ophthalmology facility that can serve the Southeast Asia region. It also plays an active role in the delivery of ophthalmologic care to underserved populations.

For more information: Asian Eye Institute, http://www.asianeyeinstitute.com.

Box 1.4 Fleury Diagnostic Center, Brazil

Founded in 1926 in Brazil, Fleury is an example of a successful network of diagnostic centers. Each day over 2,500 clients enter the doors of its 14 units in the state of São Paulo and in the cities of Brasilia and Rio de Janeiro. There they receive more than 2,000 different types of diagnostic tests, including nuclear medicine, x-rays, ultrasound, computerized tomography, magnetic resonance, mammography, and bone densitometry and histology. These tests are performed according to strict international quality standards established by organizations such as the College of American Pathologists and the ISO. To ensure that its services are available to a broad clientele, Fleury has developed partnerships with over 900 labs in Brazil.

For more information: Fleury Diagnostic Center, http://www.fleury.com.br.

---

been made to establish a network of mobile diagnostic centers that can be assembled and disassembled easily in order to visit many villages and provide diagnostic services at low cost. Some sub-Saharan countries also have successful centers for diagnosis of cancer and other diseases.

2

Project Concept and Mission Statement

The Whats and Whys of Your Project

One of the first steps to take in establishing your facility is to determine what type of institution you want to build and your rationale for doing so. These ideas should be articulated in your project concept and mission statement. These two instruments broadly define the target population you want to serve, the types of services you want to deliver, and why you believe these services are warranted. In answering these initial, critical questions, it is important always to keep in mind that your medium-size hospital (or other type of facility) will have to be financially self-sustaining. More often than not, health care facilities are developed out of a strong sense of social service with limited attention to financial sustainability or financial viability. Although altruistic motives are commendable, financial sustainability will be one of the most important defining constraints of any project, if not the most important. It is thus a crucial issue to think about early on (financial analysis is discussed in chapter 4, and obtaining financing in chapter 5).

Project Concept

Developing the concept for your hospital will be the starting point for your project. The concept should reflect your (and your partners') main motivations for building the hospital. It should address the social and business aspects of the venture and should answer, at a minimum, the following questions:

- *Why do you want to build this facility?* Do you see, for example, insufficient or inadequate facilities for medical doctors to train and practice? Do you think you could provide quality services more efficiently than existing institutions? Has the government announced a new regulation, such as allowing joint ventures between public and private hospitals, that you want to take advantage of? Do you see a good business opportunity?
- *Whom will your hospital serve?* Is the majority of your target patient population part of the local community, or are most of them foreign visitors and residents? In terms of income levels, will your hospital aim to serve low-, middle-, or high-income households?
- *What services will you provide and how will you operate?* Will your facility be a specialty clinic (such as a cancer institute or maternity facility) or a general multidisciplinary hospital? Are you providing inpatient stay only or outpatient services as well?
- *What are the financial objectives of your hospital?* Will it be a for-profit or a not-for-profit facility?

One example of a project concept would be a hospital with modest facilities that serves a low-income patient population and charges relatively low fees. In this case, the project concept would guide you to consider building a moderately equipped hospital that will not require a high level of capital investments, so as to be compatible with a lower level of revenues. At the other end of the spectrum, your objective may be to build a state-of-the-art hospital that will serve mostly foreign expatriates and tourists as well as the higher-income local population. In such case, the assumption will be that patients are able and willing to pay much higher fees, either directly or through medical plans or insurance mechanisms. Such a facility will demand much more in the way of equipment and staffing, and the level of investment necessary is likely to be of a different magnitude.

Another interesting possibility for a project concept is a facility with teaching capabilities. Such a hospital typically offers a much more sophisticated and broader range of medical services, normally to a low-income population. A teaching hospital needs to be associated with a medical school and must meet not only the needs of patients and staff but also the academic requirements of a student body and faculty. Because they must provide such a broad range of services, teaching facilities often depend heavily on large endowments and grants to sustain their operations.

If you are more concerned with providing social services than with generating profits, you might be inclined to build a hospital on a not-for-profit basis. In fact, some countries require all private health care facilities to be registered as not-for-profit entities for legal and tax purposes. On the other hand, a for-profit facility might better serve your business goals and might be managed more efficiently. Unless it has been designed with the expectation that operational losses will be covered by endowments and grants—and funding commitments have been secured prior to construction—a hospital must generate a sufficient cash flow from its operations. Any excess revenues that remain after paying for all operating costs and covering additional working capital are either plowed back fully into the facility operations in the case of a not-for-profit facility or used to pay for facility improvements, loans, interest, and dividends in the case of a for-profit facility. Therefore, the realistic distinction between a for-profit and a not-for-profit facility lies not so much in whether or not the facility needs to generate excess cash flow but rather in how the excess will be used.

After consulting practicing physicians and others who are familiar with the health sector situation in the country, you should be able to formulate the answers to the questions above. You may start out with a particular project concept that reflects your understanding at that point of how your hospital should look. However, it is very likely that your initial concept will undergo revisions as you continue your research and consultations.

Mission Statement

The mission statement articulates the project concept to the team, facility staff, patients, and outside partners. It lays out the guiding principles of your project (box 2.1). This statement should convey what the hospital is striving to become and how it intends to accomplish this. As such, it will serve as a reference point for all who are involved in the hospital's establishment and in its subsequent operating decisions and activities.

It may appear to be premature to draft a mission statement before your hospital is even built. But having this statement ready at an early stage is crucial in informing and guiding your subsequent decision making. It is important to note that many of the decisions you will make in the early planning phase of the project will have significant consequences for how the hospital will operate and evolve over the long term.

While your project concept and mission statement lay the strategic foundations for the facility that you will build, they are not set in stone. They can, and perhaps should, change over the course of the planning process.

Box 2.1 Excerpts from Sample Mission Statements

Our mission is . . .

". . . to be the premier health care facility in the region, providing acute inpatient and community-based services."
— Albury Wodonga Private Hospital, West Albury, Australia

". . . to bring health care of international standards within the reach of every individual. We are committed to the achievement and maintenance of excellence in education, research and health care for the benefit of humanity."
— Apollo Hospitals Group, Chennai, India

". . . to provide efficient world-class health care with caring and compassion. We treat our patients as we would our family members. We are prudent, honest and ethical in all our dealings. We work as a team. We continually improve the quality of everything we do. We maintain a happy environment with respect and mutual trust. We encourage professional development and innovation through a constant process of learning. We provide efficient health care to bring value to our internal and external customers."
— Bumrungrad Hospital, Bangkok, Thailand

". . . to meet and surpass our clients' expectations, ensure their full satisfaction, and make HMSL synonymous with excellence in hospital services. This means we implement a policy of total quality by integrating technology, well-being, and customer service to make HMSL a benchmark in hospital services. We count on the participation of our collaborators, physicians, and patients—from whom critical feedback and suggestions are always, welcome—to contribute in our efforts to meet completely the needs of our users."
— Hospital e Maternidade São Luiz, São Paulo, Brazil

" . . . to deliver a comprehensive first-world medical service exceeding all expectations of our valued patients."
— Reddington Hospital, Lagos, Nigeria

Project Management

As you move your project forward, the project concept and mission statement will be tested, improved, and refined through the prefeasibility and feasibility studies. The facility will be planned, designed, and constructed. Medical equipment will be bought, and the facility staffed. Financing will be secured, and marketing will build a prospective clientele. Finally, the facility will have its opening day. This process is illustrated in figure 2.1.

The top tier of the figure lays out the stages that will need to take place: project concept and mission statement, prefeasibility analysis, feasibility analysis, facility planning and design, facility construction, and facility opening. The arrow behind the stages indicates that they will occur largely in sequence, although with different levels of iteration and considerable overlap. Medical

Figure 2.1   Project Management: Establishing a Private Health Care Facility

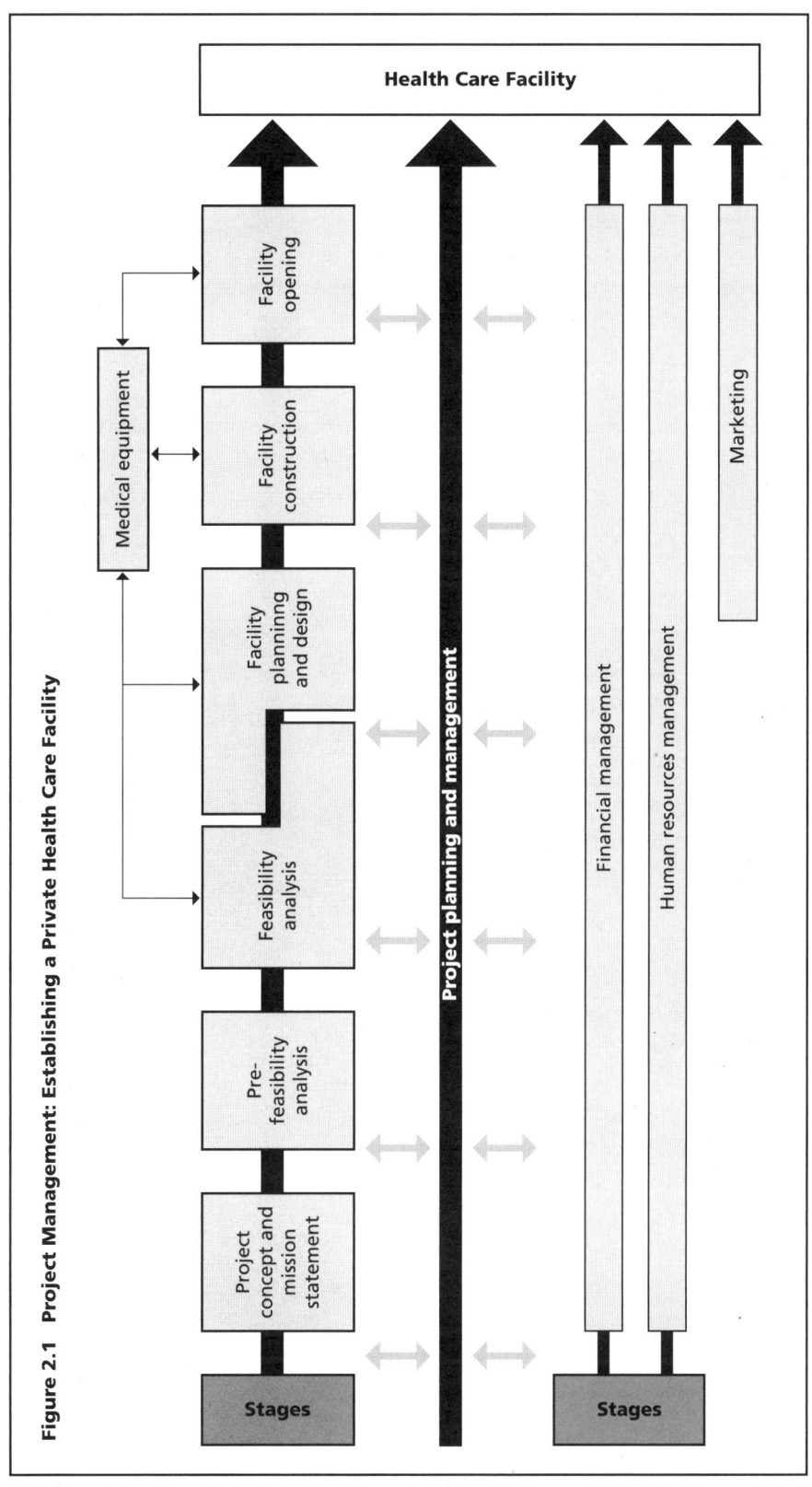

equipment is placed parallel to the sequence because activities related to medical equipment are less sequential and will take place during four of the stages: the feasibility analysis, the facility planning and design, facility construction, and facility opening. The greatest attention to medical equipment will come during the facility planning/design and construction phases.

Shown at the bottom of figure 2.1 are the major supporting functions: financial management, human resources management, and marketing. These supporting functions are essential to successful completion of the stages shown in the top part of the figure, though their complexity and intensity will vary depending on each stage of the process. The supporting functions will continue to be critically important to the hospital's operation after its opening.

In the middle of the figure, a large arrow illustrates the planning and management functions that continue throughout the project and are critical to its success. The central person who performs this role, often called the project director, provides leadership, guidance, and oversight to everyone involved in the project. The project director understands the vision and mission of the hospital and sets the priorities, standards, and key policies for the project. He or she represents the project and the project team in dealings with government agencies, architects, banks, and contractors and takes the lead role in conducting negotiations. Bringing all these pieces together is a very complex task, and will be the ultimate determinant of a project's success.

The project director is often the person who initiates the project. If you have a group of partners who have conceived the idea of developing a hospital together, you must designate one person from your group who can play this role successfully. Because this is a critical role, it requires a full-time, long-term commitment that lasts until the project is completed. In all likelihood, you and your partners, as the project initiators, will also provide the initial equity financing and thus will be called the project's owners or sponsors (these terms are used interchangeably throughout this book).

In the event that none of the partners can play the role of project director, you will have to retain a highly experienced professional to do so. The externally hired project director's loyalty and obligations will be to you and your partners. You will have to give this person a substantial level of authority to make important decisions and recommendations and to speak on behalf of the sponsors/owners in negotiations concerning all aspects of the project. However, even though you will delegate authority to the project director, there will be close interaction between the project director and your group of partners on a regular basis to ensure that you are comfortable with decisions the director will make and that there are no surprises, particularly in the areas of obtaining financing and managing cash flows.

3

The Prefeasibility Analysis

Better to Stop Now than Fail Later

Once you have defined the concept and mission statement for your hospital, the next step is to make an initial assessment of the overall potential of your concept. A prefeasibility analysis is a broad assessment of whether or not it is possible for your hospital to be built and operated the way you and your partners envision. Among other things, it seeks to uncover major risks that could seriously affect the project. Put another way, a prefeasibility analysis tests your project's viability at an early stage. If the analysis identifies a major risk that probably cannot be overcome or that would cost too much to mitigate or manage, you and your partners will be able to avoid spending valuable time and money pursuing an unworkable project.

In addition to identifying any critical risk that could jeopardize your project's viability, the prefeasibility analysis will help identify key issues that require satisfactory resolution (and determine what kind of solutions would be needed) before the project can move forward; determine what, if any, modifications to the project concept will be necessary to overcome or resolve some of the risks and issues identified; and prioritize important preparatory steps that will have substantial impact on the project's progress.

Although this assessment is an early step in the project process, it requires consideration and input related to downstream activities such as financing, marketing, and facility design. Given that it is not always easy to account for all the downstream issues at this early stage, you and your partners should expect to revise your project concept as you make progress in the prefeasibility analysis, and even during the subsequent feasibility analysis.

Conducting the Prefeasibility Analysis

You and your partners can carry out the prefeasibility analysis yourselves. If you decide to use the services of a consulting firm, you should search for an organization that has good experience relevant to your project. If you wish to retain an international consulting or advisory firm, you will need to ensure that it has a local team that is familiar with the economic, market, and regulatory environment in the country and area where your hospital will be located.

It is important to recognize that some advisers or consultants may be overly eager to affirm your views and encourage you to proceed with the project rather than to provide an objective assessment. For your own benefit, you should attempt to challenge the consultants' analysis and results before becoming too comfortable with the path chosen.

Key Questions

The following questions, among others, should be asked in the course of a prefeasibility analysis.

Does the prevailing regulatory and policy framework support the establishment of a new private facility?

It is essential to understand the national and local laws and regulations governing the establishment and operation of your hospital. At the national level, these are typically established by the ministry of health. The main aspect to be analyzed is whether or not there are any laws or regulations on the books that will make it extremely difficult for a private hospital to be built and operated or to become financially viable. If the overall legal and regulatory environment for the health care sector is focused on the public sector, there could be many constraints on the establishment of private health care facilities. It will also be important to assess, to the extent possible, ongoing or planned reforms in the health sector that could affect private provision of services.

What is the health status of the target population?

You can use demographic and health indicators to measure epidemiological trends in the health status of the country's population, as well as of the population in your target locality. Some examples of indicators that you should consider obtaining are listed in appendix D. In most countries the ministry of health publishes an annual report on health statistics, and other government departments may also issue reports on national and regional statistics related to population and health. Such reports may include information about disease prevalence and about patterns of health care provision and utilization that will help determine what type of services your hospital can offer. Health status data for many countries can also be obtained from external sources such as the World Health Organization (WHO), the Pan American Health Organization (PAHO), the World Bank Group, the United States Centers for Disease Control (CDC), the United Nations Children's Fund (UNICEF), and the United States Agency for International Development (USAID). Other sources include country-specific demographic and health surveys, as well as professional journals and reports published by industry associations and individual researchers. It will be also helpful to obtain data concerning other countries for comparison purposes.

These health indicators provide a glimpse of the overall health of a general population, but they do not tell the whole story. They often do not reveal disease-specific or locality-specific patterns that may be important to your project. In addition, the lack of reliable information for population health assessment, especially in developing countries, often prevents accurate assessment of the burden of injury and disease or the level and patterns of health care utilization. Therefore, as you collect and use data, you should keep in mind the possible gaps between the data and the reality and try to verify how valid, relevant, and recent the data may be. You will have to take into account such gaps when you prepare the plans and projections for your hospital.

Having obtained data on the underlying health sector trends in the country and region you are targeting, you should consider to what extent these trends may change in the next three to five years. What epidemiological shifts are likely to occur? How are life expectancy, lifestyles, and patterns of consumption changing—for example, as regards smoking and obesity? In light of these expected changes, will the existing medical facilities in the region or country be able to meet the population's future needs? If not, what types of additional health infrastructure and services will be required?

Is there sufficient market demand for your facility?

Market demand is a fairly broad area, covering both demand-side and supply-side factors. The characteristics of existing private and public providers, the population's demand for and capacity to pay for services, as well as the way in which health care services are paid for need to be examined. Key questions to ask at this stage include the following:

- How do most people in the target locality pay for health care?
- What percentage of population has access to health insurance?
- What fraction of annual household income on average is spent on health care, and how does this compare to the pattern in other countries?
- Is there a national health insurance plan? If there is one, does it pay for care provided by private hospitals? Is health insurance compulsory or voluntary?
- Are there private health insurance programs? Do employers provide health insurance or pay for health care provision for their employees?
- What proportion of health service payments are out-of-pocket?
- Is there public acceptance of private hospitals?
- Is health care provided by the private sector perceived to be of equal or better quality than care provided by the public sector?
- Is there excess capacity or excess demand in the health care sector? What are the main reasons for the excess capacity or demand?
- When was the last attempt to build a new hospital in the same area where your hospital will be built? Was the project successful? If it was not successful, what were primary reasons for failure?
- What, if any, types of services are clearly needed but are not being provided by existing hospitals, and why are they not provided?
- In what way is the demand for particular services likely to change over the next three to five years in view of anticipated epidemiological changes?
- How will a sizeable patient base be established? Will extensive marketing be needed? Are marketing and advertising for health care services allowed in the country?
- Are existing private facilities (hospitals, clinics, diagnostic centers, independent laboratories, and so forth) profitable? Which types of facilities are profitable and which ones are not? What are the main reasons that some are not profitable?
- How will your hospital differentiate itself from the competition?
- Are public hospitals competitors of private sector hospitals, or do the two complement one another? Are there examples of public-private partnership?
- Is the playing field even between the public and private sectors? If not, will the environment change in the next two to three years? If so, how?

How is the patient referral system structured?

In many countries, medical clinics and individual practitioners have a medical referral system in place that determines the way in which patients are directed to certain facilities for diagnostic procedures and treatments. Understanding early on how patients are referred to hospitals in the area where your hospital will be located will be one of the most critical components of your prefeasibility analysis. Joining the referral system may not be easy and can take many years depending on how the system works. Many people who are familiar with the health care industry point out that insufficient attention to this matter is one of the common causes of failure for newly constructed hospitals. It is critically important to gain a thorough understanding, at an early stage of planning, of how extensive the referral system is, how it works, and what it will take to become part of it as soon as the hospital becomes operational. This is particularly important for hospitals with foreign sponsors, or with significant proportions of foreign or expatriate physicians.

How will prices be structured, and will your target population be able to pay the prices?

In order to be financially viable, your hospital will have to charge certain prices for its services. You will need to look into the degree to which the government regulates the prices that private sector hospitals can charge. In addition, you should assess the level of market prices that would be acceptable to the public and/or your target client groups, and the extent to which your hospital will be able to increase its prices in line with inflation rates, exchange rate fluctuations, and increased costs.

The ability and willingness to pay on the part of your target population has to be carefully assessed at the same time that you address the pricing issue. This is a very difficult task, especially in countries where there are limited data available on banking and other financial services. However, if there is no national health insurance program and private health insurance programs are not well developed, the population's ability to pay for medical services would be substantially reduced. Such a situation would point to the need to develop the facility as a specialty clinic that would require less up-front investment and other resources.

How much investment will your hospital need and how will it be financed?

Even before undertaking a full feasibility analysis, it is important to get a rough idea of the project costs. Initial costs may include the purchase of land, construction of a new facility or purchase and renovation of an existing structure, purchase of equipment, marketing, and interest payments during construction.

The amount of financing that can be mobilized for your project will largely depend on the nature of your project concept and the project's expected financial viability. You will need to have initial discussions with architects and construction companies to obtain rough estimates of the project's total cost based on the project concept. Take care not to underestimate your project cost and be sure to allow for a sufficient amount of working capital and payment of interest during the first two to three years of the project, including the construction period. Obtaining a sufficient amount of equity financing will be the most challenging issue concerning financing.

How will your hospital be staffed?

It will be critically important to be able to find sufficient numbers of properly trained physicians, nurses, and technicians for your hospital. In some countries, well-trained physicians may prefer working at public rather than private hospitals even though their salaries may be lower, because of the other benefits and privileges associated with working at public hospitals. If your hospital is not going to be able to attract experienced physicians, that will have a significant impact on its operations. You should also look into the details of compensation packages that you may need to offer in order to attract qualified and well-trained physicians and nurses.

What are the key risks?

At the end of the prefeasibility stage, you will want to answer at least the following questions before deciding whether or not to proceed with the next step:

- How quickly can your hospital become a part of the patient referral system?
- Will it be possible to obtain, within a reasonable time frame, various licenses and permits necessary to build and operate your hospital (especially the hospital license)?
- Are there any important legal or regulatory restrictions that would severely limit your hospital's freedom to attract patients and set the prices it needs to charge?
- Is there sufficient market demand to justify establishing a new hospital (box 3.1)?
- Can you find a land parcel that is large enough and of suitable condition to build your hospital?
- Are there enough well-trained physicians and nurses that your hospital can hire?

Box 3.1 Challenges of Catchment and Competition

An African physician who had a successful medical practice in a Western country decided to build a 200-bed hospital in the capital city of his native country. The entrepreneur first completed a feasibility analysis and then turned to fundraising, contacting other expatriate physicians originally from the same country. It soon became clear that another physician in the diaspora, from the same relatively small African country, had earlier planned to build a 200-bed hospital and had already raised funds from some of the same people. The earlier experience did not result in any tangible output, so many of the physicians approached were reluctant to support a second effort. It was also clear that the city, which had a population of less than 1 million, would be unable to support two new high-technology hospitals opening within a couple of years of each other.

Soon after learning of the preexisting project, the physician contacted the other sponsor and began discussions of consolidating the two projects into one. Had these issues of catchment and potential competition been assessed earlier, in the prefeasibility stage, it would have saved the entrepreneur considerable expenditures for the feasibility analysis.

- Can you raise enough financing for your hospital? Most important, can you raise at least 40 percent of your estimated project cost in the form of equity financing?
- Are there any impending government decisions or other major events that could significantly affect the market situation in the next 12 to 24 months?

Risk Assessment and Management

One of the key objectives of conducting prefeasibility and feasibility analyses is to identify risks associated with the project. This section provides a brief general summary of topics related to risk assessment and risk management. It is not intended to be a comprehensive discussion of all aspects of this complex topic.

A risk can be defined as a possibility that the existence or absence of a particular fact, event, or decision could negatively affect the achievement of a desired outcome. The words "desired outcome" are key here; they signal that the risk factors are different for each party involved. Each of the parties in your project will presumably have a different definition of the outcome that they want to obtain. For example, the desired outcome for you and your partners will be construction of the hospital on time and within budget and successful operation of the facility from the social, business, and financial perspectives. Thus, you would consider as a risk the possibility of any event, activity, or decision that could jeopardize your ability to build and operate the hospital as you envision—for example, the enactment or repeal of a particular government regulation, or a business decision by a person or company. Your investors' desired outcome will include an assurance that their money will be used for the intended purposes and that they will get their money back plus an expected return on their investment within an expected time period. Any fact or event that could prevent such an outcome will be a risk factor in the eyes of an investor.

The first step is to make a comprehensive list of all the risks that you and your partners can identify and use it as a checklist. Each identified risk needs to be assessed from three perspectives: (a) how serious it is, or would be if it were to materialize; (b) how it can be quantified; and (c) how it can be managed, that is, avoided, minimized, and/or transferred to another party. The list should be specific in describing the risk as you perceive it and should specify the possible value or cost of damage that could occur if the risk becomes a reality, possible ways to mitigate the risk, the amount of time and money necessary to mitigate it, parties who might be willing to take the risk instead of you and the hospital, and so on. It is also important to give thought to how investors and other interested parties might perceive different risks associated with your project.

Social customs often influence people's perceptions of what is a risk and what is not. In assessing the seriousness of a given risk, therefore, you should consider whether social or cultural expectations may lead you to ignore a real threat to your business. For example, suppose you have two architects to choose from, both experienced. One of them has been introduced to you by a close friend of yours. However, you have also learned that this architect has a history of taking on too many projects at once and often fails to deliver the work on time. When evaluating the risk factor concerning this architect, you might think that it can be managed by asking your friend to put pressure on his friend, the architect, to give your project priority. But the results of this could be very uncertain, and so you may wish to avoid this way of looking at a risk factor.

After identifying the risks and assessing their likelihood and seriousness, you will need to assess each one in terms of the possibility of mitigation. When faced with a particular risk, most entrepreneurs will first look for an alternative way to achieve the same intended result without having to resolve the risk, thereby avoiding it. For example, say you wish to build a hospital in a country where all land is owned by the government, and thus you must lease your project site from the government. You are offered a site in a location that seems to have good growth potential, but the site needs a new, small bridge to enable people to access it. The local government is giving strong assurances, but only orally, that the bridge will be built before your hospital is constructed. If you cannot count on the local government's oral promise, you might decide to avoid the risk of the bridge not being built in time by asking for a different site to lease.

If an alternative course of action cannot be found, people will look for ways to minimize the risk factor. For example, perhaps you are planning to import major medical equipment for your hospital but you find out that the equipment manufacturer does not often send out its technicians to the country where your hospital will be located. For various reasons, you conclude that you need to buy that particular equipment and that no substitute will be suitable. Your research shows that a leading hospital in the capital city of a neighboring country has the same equipment and employs an in-house technician who has been trained by the equipment manufacturer. If you could sign an equipment service agreement with that hospital, specifying that the trained technician will service the equipment at your hospital as well, you would substantially minimize the risk of not being able to get your medical equipment repaired when the need arises.

The third way of managing a risk is to transfer it to another party. For example, after interviewing several construction companies in the area where your hospital will be constructed, you and your partners conclude that most of them seem to be in relatively weak financial condition. The country's regulations do not allow foreign construction companies to operate in the country, so your choice of a general contractor is limited. You feel that there is considerable risk that the general contractor could get into financial trouble after starting

---

Box 3.2 Protecting Your Business through Insurance

Three main types of business insurance coverage are protection of physical assets, protection of revenue, and protection against claims by third parties. It may be advantageous to insure all assets under one policy, as this may be more cost-effective and administratively easier to deal with than several different policies.

- *Protection of physical assets:* Ensure coverage of buildings (including construction), plant and equipment (including during importation), stocks of medical supplies, fixtures and fittings, office contents (including computers), motor vehicles, and any other physical assets that the business may acquire. All of these assets are at risk of being lost or damaged as a result of various perils, most of which are insurable. Perils that can be insured against include fire, lightning, explosion, flood, earthquake, storm and water damage, riot and strike, theft, and malicious damage.
- *Protection of revenue:* It is usually possible to insure for loss of revenue through coverage of either net profit and fixed expenses or fixed expenses only for the duration of any anticipated business interruption associated with loss of or damage to physical assets.
- *Protection against claims by third parties:* Any medical professional running a business is at risk of being sued for malpractice or negligence. Both the facility and the medical professionals working within the facility can be sued. The legal climate in the country and the level of consumer awareness will determine the likelihood of such claims, and also the severity of any successful legal actions or court awards. Medical malpractice insurance can be costly, and it is not always available in developing countries, but most insurers can access international markets for this. Buy coverage early, before you have any claims against the business, as once you have a history of possible claims insurance coverage will become more difficult and costly to obtain. Negotiations for this insurance should start at least three months before the facility is expected to become operational, so that there is ample time to respond to insurers' questions and to negotiate cost-effective protection.

the work on your hospital project, regardless of which of the local construction companies is selected. If this occurs and the general contractor fails to pay its workers and suppliers on time, the hospital's construction may be delayed; this will lead to delays in installation of medical equipment and other auxiliary systems, which in turn will almost certainly cause cost overruns and delay the hospital's opening. If the hospital's opening is delayed, the preopening costs will go up and, more importantly, it will take longer for the hospital to start building up its patient base and revenues. There could be other ramifications, such as a tarnished image of the hospital, the effect of which cannot be quantified or measured in monetary value. However, you can estimate the cost of delays to a reasonable degree. You may therefore decide to ask the contractor to provide you with a performance guarantee or performance bond issued by a credible bank or bonding agency. By doing so, you transfer a good part of the risk associated with a financially weak contractor to the institution that will issue the performance guarantee or bond.

You will need to identify early on the serious risks that you and your partners may find impossible to overcome or that would cost too much in time and money to mitigate, making it unrealistic or not worthwhile to try to resolve them.

As you develop contingency plans to protect your facility in the event of physical loss or damage, financial loss, or liability, you should bear in mind which risks are insurable in your local market and which are not. It is important to develop an early understanding of the local insurance market or to engage an independent broker who understands coverages available, as not all insurance products are available in all developing countries (box 3.2).

4

The Feasibility Analysis

Finding and Clearing a Path to Success

If the prefeasibility analysis indicates that the project can be viable and you decide to move forward, the next step is to conduct a detailed feasibility analysis. This examines the details of the plan throughout the facility's construction and subsequent daily operation. It should develop the specifics of how to construct and operate the hospital so as to ensure the project's feasibility and viability. You will identify and analyze the full range of risks, large and small, and determine the best ways to minimize them. In the course of the feasibility analysis, you will probably discover numerous risks that did not come to your attention during the prefeasibility stage.

The term "feasibility analysis" is often used to refer both to the *process* of analyzing a project's feasibility and to the document that is the *final output* of that process. Furthermore, the terms "feasibility analysis," "feasibility study," "project proposal," and "business plan" are often used interchangeably to refer to the final document. To keep the concepts of process and output distinct, we refer to the process of analyzing the project's feasibility as the *feasibility analysis* and to the resulting document as the *business plan*. The business plan will present all aspects of your project in detail. It has two main objectives: (a) to provide its readers with sufficient information about the project so that they can understand the project well, and (b) to convince its readers to make a positive decision to support and/or invest in the project.

In thinking through the details of your project's construction stage and subsequent daily operations, you and your partners will need to consider several different scenarios in terms of services to be offered, prices to be charged, cost-efficient ways to design and construct your hospital, ways to finance the construction and raise working capital, and so on. You will need to reach agreement on the best set of alternatives for construction, financing, and daily operation. You should consider a multistage approach, as this could provide an opportunity to grow gradually and possibly to raise financing in stages after offering proof of a viable business. Once you and your partners have come to an agreement, often with the help of experienced consultants, on the alternatives you will choose, you will prepare the business plan. The final business plan (or the final version of this document) should demonstrate clearly that your project is technically, environmentally, operationally, financially, and socially feasible. Appendix E gives an idea of the complexity of the planning that you will need to do.

Health care is often at the forefront of issues relating to economic and social development as well as poverty reduction. Increasingly, grants and technical assistance funds are being made available for activities related to health care provision. You may wish to investigate the possibility of obtaining grants to pay for the feasibility analysis and preparation of the business plan for your hospital early in the planning stage.

Conducting the Feasibility Analysis

The feasibility analysis should be conducted with an objective, realistic, and professional mindset. It is a dynamic process and requires numerous iterations as your analysis continues and your plans evolve. Often, entrepreneurs who set out to build health care facilities choose to retain an independent professional consulting firm to carry out the feasibility analysis and prepare the business plan. Should you decide to do this, you should make sure that the consultants will indeed prepare a thorough, objective, and professional analysis and will not simply seek to reinforce your desire to carry out the project.

Appendix F provides useful advice with respect to evaluating and selecting hospital consultants. In addition to elements included in the appendix, it is important to ensure that the consultants will work *with* you and your partners rather than merely work *for* you. You need to create a working relationship in which the consultant shares your vision and cares about the ultimate success of your project rather than one in which the consultant seeks only to fulfill her or his own self-interest.

You and your partners can conduct the feasibility analysis yourselves if you have sufficient knowledge, experience, and time to do so. Even so, you may need to seek advice at critical stages from someone who is not closely involved in the project but who has experience in conducting feasibility analyses, preferably in the health care sector. You may also consider undertaking certain parts of the feasibility analysis yourselves and retaining a professional firm to conduct the remaining parts of the analysis and prepare the business plan.

Whereas data for the prefeasibility analysis are gathered mainly from secondary sources, the feasibility analysis should include, as much as possible, data from both primary and secondary sources. Primary sources can include potential clients, existing hospitals, and consumer survey companies, among others. The secondary sources include reports and statistics published by government agencies, individual researchers, consulting firms, international organizations, or industry associations.

The feasibility analysis can be roughly divided into two parts, nonfinancial and financial. The nonfinancial analysis addresses key areas such as market demand, competitive landscape, macroeconomic and political environment, legal and regulatory environment, technical and technological factors, environmental and safety factors, ownership structure, organizational and management structure, and corporate governance. The financial analysis looks mainly at costs, revenues, working capital, and financing.

There is considerable overlap and interaction between the various parts of the analysis and it will not be possible to address the topics in a strict sequence. Most obviously, many choices made in the nonfinancial areas will directly affect the financial analysis. For example, the organizational and management structure helps determine staffing costs, which are a big part of the financial picture. At the same time, your analysis of the expected levels of financing and revenues will help set the parameters within which to make choices about all aspects of the hospital. For example, a hospital that expects a high level of revenues may be able to invest in more sophisticated equipment than one that anticipates a lower revenue stream.

Following are some of the basic areas to be considered in the feasibility analysis. The list is not exhaustive, and you will need to add to it according to the particularities of your project.

Nonfinancial Analysis

Market and Competitive Landscape

In order to assess whether your hospital will be viable, the market situation needs to be analyzed from the perspective of demand and supply. The following questions need to be answered fully, early in the process:

- Is there sufficient demand for the services your hospital will provide?
- Are there enough people who are willing and able to pay the prices that your hospital will need to charge in order to ensure its financial viability? Who will pay for the services and what will be the payment conditions?
- Who will be your major competitors? What would be your competitive advantage?

In the following sections, "services" and "treatments" refer only to those services and treatments that your hospital will provide.

DEMAND ANALYSIS

It is easy to become convinced that there is sufficient market demand for your services after hearing stories about how long people have to wait to receive certain treatments or how they have to go abroad for certain surgical operations. But the demand analysis must be based on more than anecdotes. In order to properly assess the level of demand, you will need to define the following aspects:

- The main catchment area, that is, the physical boundaries of the area from which 75 to 80 percent of your hospital's patients will come (for example, within 100 kilometers of the location of your facility)
- The profile of your target patients (for example, high-income, middle-income, or low-income; local population only or foreign residents as well as local population; and ethnic groups, if applicable); any particular characteristics of this population; and the estimated number of people in the target groups
- The estimated average level of health care expenses incurred annually by each family or person in the target population
- The estimated quantity or frequency of health interventions needed by your hospital's primary target patients in the main catchment area

The above questions will have been addressed during the prefeasibility analysis to a certain extent, but they should be substantially refined in the feasibility analysis.

It is important to estimate the number of inpatients and outpatients that can be accommodated at your hospital, and how large a population would be required to sustain such a patient flow. For example, a 100-bed hospital would have a total capacity of 36,500 bed-days available annually. Ideally, you should aim to achieve an 80 percent occupancy rate—often regarded as an optimum benchmark—within about three years. With an average length of stay of six days, the hospital will need about 5,000 inpatients a year to achieve 80 percent occupancy. If the hospital is located in a city of 1 million people, with a hospital admission rate of about 5 percent, it would be expected that each year about 50,000 patients would be admitted to hospitals. It will be crucial to analyze where your 5,000 paying patients will come from, the interventions they will need, and the average amount that each patient will spend at your hospital.

Whether or not 5,000 inpatients per year will be sufficient to ensure your hospital's financial viability will, of course, depend on the average revenue that can be generated from each patient, revenues from outpatient and other services, the hospital's operating expenses, and the amount of debt service required. These details can be analyzed with a well-constructed financial projection model, discussed later in this chapter.

It would be helpful if you could obtain the services of a consumer survey company, if there are companies with sufficient experience in the relevant geographical area and if you can afford their services. You could also conduct focus group discussions with medical doctors who are knowledgeable about your catchment area to find out what they see to be the major health needs of the population that you are planning to serve. Disease patterns may not be homogeneous across the population as a whole, and different diseases may affect different strata of society. If you are targeting a certain socioeconomic class, you should define the disease burden and health status of that specific group of people.

In analyzing market demand, you will need to be sensitive to people's preferences, the accessibility of the facilities, and the cultural and social aspects of the demand pattern. Cultural preferences, religious beliefs, communal and societal habits, gender differences, and a host of other factors affect people's choices in seeking out medical treatments and the ways in which they respond to these treatments.

In assessing demand, one also needs to look at structural factors. The demand for health care materializes differently from country to country depending on the structure of the health care sector, which in turn is largely driven by the government's policies and level of support. Many countries offer a national health care program and have a variety of regulations relating to administration of the program. The areas covered by the national health care program and the level of financial subsidy provided by the government often affect people's ability and willingness to seek medical treatment. In addition, research is needed to discover how the medical insurance industry is structured in the relevant country and what changes, if any, are expected in the next three to five years.

As discussed in chapter 3, you must also understand the patient referral system in place in your target markets and determine how easy or difficult it would be for your hospital to become a part of the system. What impact will this system have on your hospital's ability to attract the number of patients and generate the level of revenues it will need in order to establish its viability?

While conducting the demand analysis, you should also assess the supply side of your target market and your potential competition. A comprehensive supply analysis begins with identification of all the facilities located within your target area, as well as other facilities accessible to patients from this area. In order to be able to visually analyze the level of supply, it is helpful to prepare a map with the location and size of each hospital indicated. Such a map can also illustrate aspects such as accessibility by public transportation that affect each hospital's competitive edge.

Your list should include key information about each facility, such as number of years in operation, reputation, number of departments, number of beds by department or by type, number of operating rooms, services offered and prices charged, quality of facilities, key medical equipment, main catchment area, how many patients are treated at the hospital each year, bed occupancy rates and trends over recent years, average waiting time for certain treatments or procedures, number of surgical operations by type of operation, capacity and utilization rate of key equipment, numbers of physicians and nurses, where the hospital's physicians come from, the hospital's business model, accessibility by public and private transportation, public or private ownership, for-profit or not-for-profit status, affiliation with a religious or other type of organization, ownership structure, quality of management, expansion plans, and so on.

This research should cover any new facilities that are either in construction or in the planning stage, as long as there is sufficient basis to expect that they will be operating in your main catchment area within the next 12 to 24 months. It is also important to analyze the expected growth in capacity and other supply trends in markets relevant to your hospital, and to understand the forces underlying these trends.

Having prepared a comprehensive list of existing facilities, you will be able to assess the existing supply capacity for the services you want to offer and compare it to the level of demand that you have estimated. This analysis should lead to a reasonable conclusion as to whether or not there is sufficient excess demand for the services you plan to offer—that is, demand that is not being met by existing hospitals and that is unlikely to be met by any new hospitals scheduled to open.

In analyzing the supply side, it is important to consider alternative health care services used by the population of the country and particularly by the population in your target markets. Use of alternative health care, including religious or traditional practices, is likely to vary depending on a population's ethnicity and socioeconomic status.

PRICING

You will need to determine the prices that would be both acceptable and affordable to the patients that your hospital will target. The process of developing the prices that your hospital will charge for its services should have started during the prefeasibility analysis period. Therefore, when you start the feasibility analysis, you will most likely finalize the pricing table for each treatment or procedure that your hospital will offer. It is possible that you may not have the full information necessary to determine prices for some procedures or treatments in the early stage of this process. You should therefore establish provisional prices for these, run the financial projections using the provisional numbers, and finalize the prices before completing the feasibility analysis. Note that pricing needs to be updated even after the hospital has started operation.

Your pricing decisions will depend on such factors as (a) prices charged by competitors; (b) prices mandated by government regulations; (c) the target population's income levels and their willingness and ability to pay; (d) capital and operating costs of your hospital; (e) the mix of payment types (out-of-pocket, publicly financed insurance, or privately financed insurance); and (f) the image and reputation of your hospital, which will influence people's willingness to pay. Pricing will be one of the most critical determinants of the demand for your hospital's services, and yet it will be very difficult to obtain the information necessary to make well-informed decisions.

Some of the above-noted aspects of pricing are mutually dependent. For example, the hospital's ability to charge certain prices will depend in part on the image and reputation that the hospital establishes, especially in the early days after it starts up operations. But its image and reputation will in turn be affected by the prices that are charged. A similar relationship exists between high capital cost and pricing.

Several of the pricing factors, such as the capital cost and image of the facility, are internally driven factors that are largely under your control. But these can provide only a partial basis for your pricing decisions. Externally driven, market-based factors must also be taken into account. When evaluating information on prices charged by other hospitals, be sure to make adjustments to reflect differences between the existing hospitals and your planned hospital. The differences could include diversity of services, quality of facilities and services, and reputation. In some developing countries, hospitals charge separate fees for diagnostic services such as x-rays, for meals, and even for fresh bed linens, so the total cost to the patient often exceeds what is presented as the price for a particular surgical procedure and/or hospitalization.

When you seek out pricing information from other hospitals, it is helpful to obtain information not only from the hospitals operating in your target area but also from those located in other cities in the country. You may also want to consider the prices charged by hospitals in other countries, especially those that patients from your target area are known to travel to for treatments. Many hospitals now publish their prices (at least their standard prices) on their Web sites. In many countries, bundling a set of services and charging one price for the package, rather than separate prices for each service, has become quite common. For example, Bumrungrad Hospital in Bangkok, Thailand, offers package prices for a variety of procedures and services and publishes them on its Web site. If you choose to adopt that type of pricing policy, you will still need to identify the individual components of the bundle of services, cost them separately, and price them separately before determining a price for the package. This is to ensure that you are fully aware of the potential impact of such a pricing practice on your hospital's financial performance.

Having obtained data for comparable services from potential competitors, you will need to verify the appropriateness of the prices you plan to charge by carrying out a projected costing sheet for each of the key revenue generators. For this purpose, you will project various costs and expenses of each organizational unit that your hospital will have and establish a basis for allocation of costs to each category of treatments or procedures. You will essentially create a miniature income statement for each of the major revenue-generating items (treatments or procedures) for each major profit center, and compute the estimated cost of each procedure or treatment. You then add the desired profit margin to obtain the prices you will need to charge in order to be able to ensure the hospital's financial viability. These cost-based prices should be compared to the prices obtained after making necessary adjustments to the pricing data obtained from other hospitals.

In addition to all the factors noted above, your hospital's ability to charge the prices desired will depend in part on how good your marketing strategy is and how well it is implemented. Marketing is discussed in more detail in chapter 6.

PAYMENT SYSTEM

The way in which you will collect payments for your services will depend on what type of insurance system, if any, exists in the country where your hospital will be located. Many developing countries have publicly funded national health insurance systems, some of which control pricing and supply of services. These systems are often underfunded, and as a result, significant payment delays may be a chronic problem. Aside from public health insurance systems, other sources of payment include private insurance and out-of-pocket payments by households, or a combination thereof. You should also assess both the likelihood of delays in payments from insurance systems—or refusal to pay for certain types of procedures—and the willingness and ability of individuals to pay for private services, if out-of-pocket spending is prevalent.

Along with the sources of payment, forms of pricing and payment also differ. There are four common methods by which private hospitals receive payments (see appendix G).[8] Under fee for service, payment is made per individual item of service. With case payment, the payment is for a package of services or an episode of care; for example, fees may be predetermined based on particular diagnosis-related groups (DRGs). Providers paid by this mechanism tend to focus on improving efficiency, which is often reflected in a reduced average length of stay for hospital inpatients. Under a per diem arrangement, a flat charge is billed for each day of hospitalization and care. Finally, with a contracting arrangement there is an agreed payment for a selected group (or all) services in a given period.

YOUR HOSPITAL'S COMPETITIVE POSITION

Once you have determined that there is sufficient demand for the services you plan to offer, you will need to assess each competitor's strengths and weaknesses as well as anticipated changes, if any, in the competitive position of each hospital that could diminish the chances of success for your hospital. This analysis will provide you with an assessment of your hospital's competitive position in your key target markets. The analysis needs to cover quantitative elements as well as qualitative and descriptive aspects. For each competitive strength and weakness identified, you should consider what actions or events could possibly weaken the strong areas or strengthen the weak areas. This exercise should be done for each of your hospital's potential competitors as well as for your own hospital. You will need to document this analysis in as much detail as possible to serve as a reference for the future. You should also include it in the business plan for your hospital.

Macroeconomic and Political Environment

People's spending patterns are influenced by overall economic conditions and trends. An overview of the broad political and economic environment in the country and your target region is an essential part of the feasibility analysis. In addition to examining the current situation, you will also review the trends over the past few years and project trends a few years into the future, seeking to

---

8. World Health Organization, *Evaluation of Recent Changes in the Financing of Health Services: Report of a WHO Study Group*, WHO Technical Report Series No. 829 (Geneva: World Health Organization, 1993).

identify the dynamics that could cause significant changes in the overall environment. The government's economic, fiscal, and monetary policies at the macro and micro levels have substantial effects on people's choices and consumption patterns. Moreover, any discernible political uncertainties in the country will likely influence the decisions of potential partners and investors. The following questions, among others, should be asked:

- What is the outlook for overall economic growth in the country and your hospital's catchment area for the next three to five years?
- What drives economic growth nationally and regionally in your hospital's target market area? What is the outlook for the economic drivers, that is, key industries, in the country and in the region?
- What is the annual per capita income in the country and in your hospital's target market area? What is the outlook for growth in per capita income?
- Is the health care sector a priority area for government spending? What are the possible changes in government priorities in the next few years?
- What are key features of the government's monetary policy? Is the government planning to relax the money supply by decreasing the central bank reserve rates for commercial banks, or vice versa? Is the government expected to lower or increase interest rates in the near future? What will be the time frame for any action in that regard?
- What has been the inflation rate nationally and regionally in the past three to five years? What are expected changes in inflation in the next three to four years? How would the anticipated inflation rate changes affect capital and operating costs of your project?
- What are official exchange rates for major hard currencies? Are they close to market rates? If not, how large are the gaps between the two? How stable have the official and market exchange rates been in the past three to five years? If the exchange rate has been stable in recent years, is any change expected in the near future? What are the chances for a sudden devaluation of the local currency?
- How stable is the political climate? How will a change in government affect the sustainability and profitability of your facility? On average, how long do health ministers stay in power?
- What political forces might influence the operations of your facility, including the choice of services to be provided by it?
- How will the existence of, or potential for, corruption in the country affect your ability to conduct business?

Legal and Regulatory Environment

The legal and regulatory framework of the country and the local area relevant to your project will have a large impact on how your hospital can be established and operated. Research should include not only existing laws and regulations but also policy papers, government circulars, and other documents that may be relevant to the health care sector.

If the country's laws and regulations and the policy positions of the government tend to change frequently, this instability could mean a higher risk for your project. In addition, sometimes the manner in which laws and regulations are interpreted and enforced can be inconsistent and irregular, and this will pose an additional risk. Therefore, you will need to assess the stability of the legal and regulatory environment at the national and regional levels. Try to find out what new laws and regulations are expected to come into effect and when, and how they could affect your project.

Key areas of the legal and regulatory landscape are examined in more detail below. Following are a few general questions to guide your research:

- How often do regulations relating to health care (including the pharmaceutical sector) change? Are substantial reforms pending?
- How feasible is it to work within the constraints of local government regulations?
- Is there any regulation concerning capacity (number of institutions, beds, etc.)?
- What are the regulations concerning treatment of emergency patients?
- Are there regulations that affect patient referrals by physicians?
- Is there any requirement that private health care facilities provide free services?
- What kinds of licenses and permits will be needed to operate your facility? What regulations govern the issuance (and revocation) of such licenses and permits? What are costs related to obtaining such licenses and permits?
- Do physicians have a choice in where they can practice?
- Are hospitals allowed to take out loans?
- Does the government subsidize payments for private health care?
- What regulations, if any, affect the choice and procurement of major medical equipment?

LAWS AND REGULATIONS GOVERNING THE HEALTH CARE SECTOR

Licensing, accreditation, and certification are the most commonly used approaches to regulating the market entry of health care businesses and the quality of health care provided. Licensing aims to ensure that health care facilities will meet certain minimum standards. Licenses are also required for physicians, nurses, and technicians. Since licenses aim to ensure the quality of health care services, renewal is required at regular intervals following confirmation that the facilities and individuals continue to meet the standards set by the regulating authorities. In almost all countries licenses are granted by government authorities.

Unlike licensing, accreditation and certification are usually carried out by independent nongovernmental organizations (NGOs), usually professional accreditation agencies or professional associations such as the Joint International Commission (box 4.1). They examine and approve the technical adequacy of health care facilities, aspects of the health care facilities' operations, as well as individual practitioners. In some countries, government also controls the standards of accreditation, in which case the accreditation service is provided either by a government agency or by a quasi-government entity that combines the expertise of public institutions and private sector professionals.

In addition to medical licensing and accreditation, permits may be needed for other aspects of your hospital's operation, including dispensing of controlled substances and handling of food. There may also be other restrictions or requirements that exist in practice due to decisions made by nongovernmental entities, such as national physicians' associations. Obtaining the various licenses and permits for a new hospital is often a complex and time-consuming process.

Box 4.1 Accreditation of Health Care Organizations: JCAHO and JCI

The Joint Commission on Accreditation of Health Care Organizations (JCAHO) is a nonprofit organization that sets standards and evaluates and accredits health care organizations and health care programs in the United States. JCAHO standards pertain to a health care organization's ability to provide safe, high-quality care and to the organization's level of performance in key functional areas. As the largest accreditor of health care organizations in the United States, JCAHO surveys nearly 20,000 health care programs through a voluntary accreditation process. JCAHO is governed by a 29-member board of commissioners experienced in health care, business, and public policy. Its corporate members include the American College of Physicians, the American College of Surgeons, the American Dental Association, the American Hospital Association, and the American Medical Association.

Joint Commission International (JCI) is a division of Joint Commission Resources, a subsidiary of JCAHO. JCI provides international accreditation and education/consultation services to other countries. Some hospitals are interested in JCI or other types of accreditation because of the focus on quality and the perceived benefits for marketing. It may take up to three years from the time of the initial request to receive accreditation from JCI.

For more information: Joint Commission on Accreditation of Health Care Organizations, http://www.jointcommission.org/, and Joint Commission International, http://www.jointcommissioninternational.com/.

It requires meticulous preparations and persistent follow-up until the necessary documents have been secured.

Regulations may affect price setting and reimbursement mechanisms in the health sector, as discussed above. The government may set direct limits on prices for particular procedures or for hospital room charges, and/or on third-party payments.

LAWS AND REGULATIONS CONCERNING FINANCING

In some countries, health care facilities are not allowed to incorporate as business entities with their own legal identities or to operate on a for-profit basis. Such rules usually mean also that a health care facility cannot take out loans in its own name. If the country in which your hospital will operate has such regulations, you will need to find the best way to build the hospital and conduct business consistent with local regulations. You will most likely need to consult experienced lawyers and financial consultants on such matters.

LAWS AND REGULATIONS CONCERNING FOREIGN INVESTMENT

Because almost all developing countries have a shortage of capital, most have regulations concerning foreign investment, affecting both loan and equity capital. Some countries offer incentives to attract foreign capital while others impose restrictions on it, particularly on foreign currency loans. Some of the incentives and/or restrictions may apply to private health care facilities such as your project. You should be fully familiar with the local regulations concerning foreign capital, both loan and equity, before contacting potential foreign financial partners for your hospital project. Your research should include (but not be limited to) the importation of foreign capital, foreign ownership of businesses and companies, foreign ownership of real property including land and buildings, repatriation of equity capital, repayment of foreign currency loans, payment of dividends, and taxes related to all such matters.

LAWS AND REGULATIONS CONCERNING STAFFING AND EMPLOYMENT

Because of the potential impact on public health, staffing of health care facilities is subject to various regulations set by governments in many countries. To begin with, there is the need to confirm the technical qualifications of medical staff through the existence of valid licenses.

The following questions, among others, should be asked in relation to staffing and employment:

- Are physicians and nurses allowed to work in both the public and private sectors at the same time? Do they have a choice in reality as to where they practice?
- What restrictions govern the hiring and laying off of employees in general and employees in the health care sector in particular, and how will these restrictions affect your ability to create the best staffing arrangement for your facility?
- Are health care personnel allowed to form unions in the country where your hospital will operate? If so, what has been the trend in the working relationships between medical personnel unions and health care institutions in recent years?
- What regulations exist concerning work hours, employee safety, mandatory training, and so forth, for health sector employees?
- What regulations exist concerning wages? Are there mandatory employee benefits, and if so, how will they affect your costs?
- Can you hire foreign staff, especially foreign medical staff, if necessary? What regulations, including those related to licensing, taxes, and payments, govern the hiring of foreign medical staff? Are there restrictions on foreign-exchange repatriation of foreign staff salaries? Are any new regulations anticipated within the next 12 to 24 months?

Laws and Regulations Concerning Agreements and Contracts

You will need to enter into numerous agreements in the course of planning for and establishing your hospital. As part of the feasibility analysis, necessary contracts should be listed and grouped by type and/or subject. Possible types of agreements include the following (you will not necessarily need all the agreements on the list, and you may need others not included here):

- Agreements for legal advisory services, financial advisory services, and accounting services
- Agreement for leasing of office space for use by the project team during the planning and preopening stages
- Agreement for the purchase or lease of land
- Agreements for obtaining services from architects, a construction manager, a general construction contractor, and subcontractors if necessary
- Agreements with specialized consultants such as a medical planner, medical equipment planner, and project manager

- Agreements for procurement of medical and nonmedical equipment and supplies, including drugs and other pharmaceutical supplies
- Agreement for procurement of an information technology system
- Agreements with insurance companies and/or a national health care insurance fund, if applicable
- Agreements with physicians for patient referral services, if applicable
- Agreements with physicians and medical and nonmedical employees
- Agreements with equity investors
- Agreements with lenders
- Agreements for technical assistance or hospital management, if applicable

In addition to full-scale contracts, a letter of intent, memorandum of understanding, or letter of commitment can formalize certain types of agreements. To protect your rights and minimize any potential liabilities, you must retain experienced legal adviser(s) and consult the adviser(s) on all matters concerning the various legal contracts and quasi-legal documents. Depending on the identity of the parties involved, some agreements may fall under the jurisdiction of a locality and/or country other than the ones where your hospital will be located. You should understand the basics of the legal framework concerning various agreements and contracts in all relevant jurisdictions.

REGULATIONS CONCERNING TRADE AND TAXES

The following questions are among those you will need to ask about trade and taxes:

- What types of taxes and quasi-taxes will your project have to pay in connection with income, staff salaries, purchase of equipment and supplies, and so on? How are these tax regulations enforced?
- What types of import tariffs are in place and how will they affect the procurement of medical equipment, drugs, and other supplies?
- How exactly does the customs clearance process work? Are there typically delays in this process, or are there other customs issues that could affect your project's completion and operations?
- What kinds of incentives are available for private health care facilities—for example, tax exemptions, duty exemptions, reduced utility charges, land for free or at discounted prices, low-interest rate loans, and so on? Are there any direct subsidies for private health care facilities?

REGULATIONS CONCERNING ENVIRONMENTAL AND OCCUPATIONAL SAFETY MATTERS

The feasibility analysis should examine the implications of all relevant national and local regulations concerning such matters as water quality, management of medical and nonmedical wastes, hazardous materials management, and worker safety. For comparison purposes and to prepare for meeting the requirements of international investors, you should also obtain and study various standards set by the United Nations, the European Union, the World Health Organization, the World Bank, and other international organizations. You can look into the availability of grants and technical assistance funds that may be available for this purpose.

OTHER REGULATIONS

There may be other regulations that could affect the way in which your hospital can be established and operated. The review of national laws on health care that you undertake near the beginning of this process may point you toward other areas of relevant regulation.

Technical and Physical Factors

The feasibility analysis should consider whether or not the construction of necessary buildings and auxiliary facilities can be completed according to the architectural plan and at an affordable cost. All elements relevant to construction of the facilities, including the location and condition of the site, the quality of construction companies available, the availability of construction materials, the timing of obtaining various permits, and so forth, must be examined. Attention should be paid to the sequence of steps, the assignment of responsibilities, and the time and costs involved in each aspect of construction, as well as any risks that may affect this process.

SITE SELECTION

The timing of land acquisition necessary for your hospital will need to be considered carefully. Ideally, you will identify an appropriate site for your hospital early in the process and obtain a strong contractual commitment from the owner of the land to either sell or lease it to you for your hospital.

In an urban area, a plot of land large enough for a hospital may not be available easily or it may be very costly if it is available. In deciding on the size of the land parcel to be acquired, you should take into account the potential for future expansion of your facility as well as the possible need for additional parking space as car ownership rises over the years. In countries where private ownership of land is allowed, the process of negotiating a purchase with the landowner will probably focus mainly on the price of the land, assuming that the historical use of the land (for example, agriculture land or landfill) can be confirmed.

In many developing countries, the government offers plots of government-owned land located in special development zones for construction of schools and hospitals. Negotiating terms and conditions with government agencies for the purchase or lease of government-owned land can be time-consuming and complicated. In such cases, you may need to allow extra time for conclusion of the land purchase or lease agreement (or land-use rights agreement) with relevant government agencies.

In addition to size, considerations in site selection include the condition of the land, its boundaries, its location, and access to roads, power, potable water lines, and a sewage system. The condition of the soil should be tested before the land is purchased or leased to uncover potential environmental problems or construction difficulties. For example, if the land was used for landfill in the past, contaminated soil could cause problems for your project. The location of the land should be assessed in terms of its vulnerability to natural disasters such as earthquake, flood, or landslide. If the site is near a swamp or a river, you might also need to consider the possible impact of rising water levels due to global warming.

If there is any reason for concern about the condition of the land, and if an alternative piece of land cannot be found, the preferred course of action would be to demand that the seller take, at the seller's own cost, corrective actions necessary to allow the construction of a hospital. In many cases, sellers may not wish to undertake costly remedies; when the seller is a government agency, bureaucratic procedures could stand in the way of such actions. In such cases the seller may be willing to accept a lower price in exchange for transferring to the buyer the responsibility of remediation. You need to ensure that the potential problems are indeed remediable at an affordable cost before deciding to accept the risks related to potential problems with the land. Some risks may be too high to justify purchase of the land even at a lower price.

You should also take into account other facilities that exist near the site, in terms of both their potential impact on your hospital and your hospital's potential impact on them. This assessment should include industrial projects that are in the planning stages as well as those already built. For example, if there is a plan to build a large pollution-emitting chemical plant near your hospital's site, you will need to consider its potential impact on the image of your hospital and the reactions from potential patients and employees before deciding to choose the site. This is why you need to know about the plans of all relevant government agencies and departments—not just health-related agencies or departments—before deciding on the site.

Another consideration is how your patients will get to the hospital and how easily ambulances can reach the hospital in case of emergency. If the hospital is going to target mainly middle- and low-income households, the question of accessibility is particularly important because most clients will rely on public transportation. Often new projects are built in special development zones that are developed without adequate roads and bridges. Even when a main road exists, an access road may not exist, so the project ends up building the access road at its own cost.

The terms and conditions of the land purchase or lease agreement or land-use rights agreement should include key aspects such as:

- Warranties for the title of the land
- Warranties for suitability of the land for hospital construction
- Preparation of the land (for example, land filling) at seller's cost before handover
- Corrective actions to remedy any existing environmental problems, if applicable, to be taken by the seller at seller's cost
- Access to utility lines and sewage facilities
- Key milestones for handover
- Rights of the buyer to conduct geotechnical tests and actions to prepare the land for construction, if needed
- Payment terms, cancellation conditions, terms for refund of deposits, and so forth.

Such agreements can be quite complicated, depending on the circumstances, and you will need the advice of experienced lawyers. You should also verify proper documentation of the land title and conduct due diligence on any pending lawsuits or disputes regarding the site before signing any agreement or making payments.

If you do not have sufficient funds to purchase all the land that you deem necessary for future expansion, you can sometimes acquire a land purchase option for the additional plot. You can buy such an option (effective, say, for five to 10 years) by entering into a land purchase option agreement with the landowner and paying a price for the option. The option rights can also be incorporated into the land purchase or lease agreement instead of being subject to a separate agreement. If you are going to lease the land, you might consider including a right to buy the land before the end of the leasing period. The terms and conditions of the option agreement should be carefully structured and negotiated so that your option rights cannot be canceled without your consent.

FACILITY PLANNING AND DESIGN

In the early stage of planning, you and your partners will form a core team to discuss the physical setting of the hospital, its design and infrastructure, and many other details. This team should include your chief executive officer or medical planner (see chapter 7), the medical equipment planner (also see chapter 7), the architect, the construction manager (if available), and the director of nursing. The role of a construction manager is uncommon in many developing countries but is a very important one (see chapter 9 for discussion of the construction manager's role).

The process of designing a hospital is often done with a "supply-side" perspective. That is, architects work with an eye to what is deemed good architecture or what will facilitate construction, but with insufficient attention to functionality of design, such as the ease of movements of patients and staff (box 4.2). Instead, the hospital should be designed to suit the services it will provide and the profile of the majority of patients who will use it.

The choice of a design for the hospital, the materials required, and the availability of locally made materials will affect total project cost and construction time. For this reason, you will need to involve an experienced construction manager (or potential construction contractor if a construction manager is not available) during the design stage so that you can benefit from his or her advice on various cost-saving measures.

It is likely that the architectural plans will undergo numerous revisions as the feasibility analysis and other research continue. Sometimes the initial decision on the choice of services to be provided by the hospital will change as the project's planning progresses. For this reason, your estimates of construction costs will vary depending on different scenarios of the services to be provided and the hospital's design. It will be useful to hold early discussions with your core construction team members on ways to minimize the number of revisions to the architectural plan.

Box 4.2   The Importance of Design Functionality

When O. A., a physician-entrepreneur, decided to build a hospital in a West African country, he contracted the services of a respected architectural firm known for building hotels in the area. However, the firm's lack of experience in hospital design kept its architects from creating an appropriate hospital layout. According to O. A., when he showed the designs to a well-known Indian architect who had designed several health care facilities in India and Sri Lanka, he was told that his architects had designed a "hotel for patients." Reluctant to enlist the services of another local architectural company, O. A. decided to deal with the problem by sending the team of architects to spend two weeks with the architects in India. He describes the two-week learning experience as an "expensive but necessary step for building a well-designed health care facility."

Information Technology Factors

Information technology (IT) requirements often take the form of a management information system package. A properly designed and installed management information system/hospital information system (MIS/HIS) is critical to smooth and efficient operation of the hospital and collection of critical data. It will allow the hospital to integrate data inputs and information outputs that include, among other things, patient data, physician's notes, pharmacy operation, billing, accounts receivable, inventory management, and the production of financial statements.

There are not many providers of integrated MIS/HIS packages for hospitals, and fewer still who offer their services to projects in developing countries. Existing software packages can be customized, but if this is not done carefully, it can create a substantial burden in terms of maintenance and continuous modification. Some experts believe that it is better to develop a hospital's information collection and generation functions and procedures around an MIS/HIS package that has been used by many other hospitals, thus avoiding a newly developed system that has not been tested by others. Customizing an MIS/HIS package, even when done by the vendor, is time-consuming and costly and will require the medical director, nursing director, chief financial officer, and other key members of your hospital's management team to work closely with the MIS/HIS package provider. In order to be able to make the right decisions about modification of the vendor's standard MIS/HIS package, you will need an IT manager who is fully knowledgeable about the issues involved in procuring and installing an MIS/HIS, or who at least knows where to find help if it is needed.

A well-developed MIS/HIS package can cost $1 million or even more. Therefore, you will need to start the search for an IT package supplier early in the feasibility analysis and obtain realistic price quotations that cover all activities needed for smooth launching of the system. Further information related to procurement and installation of an MIS/HIS is provided in chapter 10.

Environmental and Safety Factors

You will need to start preparing a draft policy and procedures manual for handling of environmental and patient and worker safety issues at an early stage. During the feasibility analysis, you will address issues such as how medical wastes will be disposed of and/or treated, safe handling of various industrial gases, safe handling of blood, disposal of laboratory materials and supplies, and radiology safety. You will need to identify major risks concerning these matters and prepare an action plan that meets international requirements. Documenting the discussions in the early stage will save time and effort later on in developing the hospital's written policies and procedures for environmental and safety issues.

Ownership Structure

During the feasibility analysis, you will consider what type of ownership structure would be most suitable for the facility you are planning to build. The answer will depend on multiple factors, beginning with the type and scale of the planned facility and whether the project will be for-profit or not-for-profit. You need to determine the amount and timing of capital needed, particularly equity capital, and ask what types of investors will participate in the project. How many key people are involved in the early stage of conceptualizing and financing the preparatory period? Will they provide equity capital for the project? Do they want to become owners of the project?

You should also consider what ownership structure would provide the required flexibility if the facility should need to expand in the future, with a corresponding expansion of the capital structure. Various tax and accounting regulations must be taken into account, along with other legal and regulatory limitations on ownership of a health care facility in your country. Another consideration is the need to minimize the exposure of investors and founding partners to liabilities potentially arising from the project.

A summary description of three common forms of ownership is provided in appendix H.

Organization and Management Structure and Staffing

During the feasibility analysis, you need to start developing the details of how the hospital will be managed after it begins operation, including the overall organizational structure, the management team, corporate governance, and staffing.

MANAGEMENT AND STAFFING

The first step is preparation of an organizational chart that shows the structure of the hospital's decision-making body and management. You should consider how to identify members of the management team, such as the medical director, the nursing director, the chief finance officer, and so forth.

In many developing countries, a shortage of well-trained medical professionals, especially those with administrative skills, is a serious impediment to

> **Box 4.3   Physician Shortage Limits Services**
>
> A physician-entrepreneur in a central African country built an 80-bed hospital in the country's largest city. The plan was for a secondary care hospital that would provide specialist services. However, the country had very few specialist physicians in residence. For certain important specialties such as cardiology, there was only one qualified physician in the country. The entrepreneur decided to bring in specialist physicians from South Africa to work full time at the hospital, but he soon realized that the cost of such a venture was prohibitive and that it would be difficult to retain these physicians over long periods of time. He then decided to change the model by hiring the South African specialists on weekends only. As a result, the hospital could not offer services in certain specialty areas on weekdays, which significantly limited the level of these services as well as the income they could generate. This case demonstrates the importance of thinking through staffing issues before deciding what type of services will be offered by the hospital.

development of new health care facilities. It may be possible to recruit expatriates to fill certain key positions on the management team. However, relying substantially on foreign medical and management staff (either individuals or corporations) can be risky. Health care is an inherently local business, and its success is determined in part by how well the project's sponsors understand local systems and preferences. Foreign individuals or companies may be unfamiliar with local business practices, cultural differences, and social customs. If your hospital is going to need to hire foreign managers, physicians, and nurses, you must pay close attention to how well the expatriates and local staff work together, as well as to the cost implications of hiring foreign staff.

Medical staff is the single most important component in any health care facility. A strong and dedicated team of well-qualified practitioners is a critical differentiator in any hospital's ability to build up and sustain a good reputation. It will also be a key factor in allowing your hospital to gain a sustainable advantage in a competitive health care market. Therefore, your ability to attract and retain the required medical and technical staff will be a critical success factor for your project (box 4.3).

You should identify where your physicians will come from and under what type of employment or service agreement they will be hired. In some countries and regions, private hospitals rely heavily on physicians who have regular jobs at public hospitals but also practice at private hospitals on a part-time basis. The efficiency and sustainability of such an arrangement must be analyzed carefully and an alternative staffing plan may be necessary to improve the project's viability.

CORPORATE GOVERNANCE

If you plan to incorporate the hospital as a limited liability company (see appendix H), you will need to consider the structure of the board of directors and an appropriate policy for corporate governance, public disclosure of key information on the hospital and its operations, and other matters. The importance of ensuring good corporate governance is to demonstrate that the hospital's highest authority makes decisions in a professional and transparent way.

INTERNAL CONTROL

An effective internal control system helps to prevent or minimize the possibility of fraud, theft, and/or poor handling of cash, important documents, supplies, equipment, and so on. It entails well-developed procedures for handling information separately from handling of cash and materials (this is why the availability of a good management information system is important). A good internal control system will also help ensure efficiency in day-to-day operations and contribute to a good working capital management system that minimizes the amount of outstanding working capital.

TRAINING

The feasibility analysis should take into account the level and type of training and the timing and cost of training programs that will be necessary for the hospital's staff. Such costs should be reflected in the financial projections. You can look into the possibilities of obtaining grants or subsidies that might support training of your staff, as well as ways to join another hospital's staff for training programs to reduce costs. The business plan should document the policies and procedures for special and regular staff training programs.

OUTSOURCING MANAGEMENT

Sometimes project developers in developing countries realize that they will not be able to mobilize the manpower and management skills needed to operate the hospital properly, so they consider the possibility of outsourcing. There are not many hospital management chains in the world and even fewer operate in developing countries. Therefore, finding a reliable management company that can take over the full responsibility of operating the hospital is likely to prove very difficult. More often, a project will contract a consulting company for a limited period of time to carry out specified tasks, as it is usually possible to hire well-qualified and experienced foreign individuals for specific functions. It is important to find the right person who can add value to your team and work harmoniously with your staff. Cultural and language differences are often a problem.

Financial Analysis: No Margin, No Mission

The main purpose of conducting a financial viability analysis is to determine whether or not the project will be able to generate enough cash from its operations over a certain time period to pay for (a) all of its operating costs; (b) debt service, that is, repayment of loan principal and interest charges and fees; (c) capital expenditures that will be needed on an ongoing basis once the facility begins operating; and (d) dividends and other forms of return on equity and quasi-equity financing. Therefore, the financial analysis should answer two critical questions. First, does it make financial sense to build and operate the hospital in the way that is being considered? And second, what conditions are required to ensure that the hospital can operate on a positive cash-generating basis?

Often, physicians and medical entrepreneurs yield to the temptation of trying to build a state-of-the-art hospital without due regard for its financial viability. As a result, either the hospital is built but gets into financial difficulty not long after opening its doors to the public, or it ends up half-completed and unable to deliver the services it was intended to provide.

During the prefeasibility analysis and the early stage of the feasibility analysis, you are likely to work with rule-of-thumb estimates for the total cost of your project. The most common method is to make a rough estimate of cost per bed—typically $100,000 to $350,000 per bed, excluding the cost of land, but it will vary depending on the location and style of the hospital and the type of services it will offer. For example, if you and your partners start with an idea for a 100-bed secondary care hospital, you might begin with an estimated total cost of $10 million to $35 million, excluding the cost of land. As you begin to firm up your plans for the hospital, you will prepare a rough budget for the entire project by major cost item. A sample format for project cost estimation is provided in appendix I.

The cost estimates need to be prepared in terms of quarterly or at least half-yearly intervals. This will provide you with the basis for preparing the financing plan. When you estimate project costs and the financing plan, keep in mind that the physical implementation and cash payouts will occur at different times. The amounts and timing of cash payments will depend on the contractual arrangements you enter into at various stages of the project and will not necessarily reflect the scope of progress being made in construction or installation.

Therefore, you should prepare the quarterly or annual project cost estimates and the financing plan from a cash flow perspective. This will help you better manage your cash flow, which is critically important. It will also help you realistically estimate financing costs, that is, the amounts of fees and interest payments that will come due during the construction period. Both of these aspects will help you avoid a cash shortfall.

As discussed below, it is important to prepare the financial projection model at an early stage of the feasibility analysis. You can use the projection model as an interactive tool to test the financial impact of several alternative scenarios and determine the most realistic and affordable choices for construction and financing. As discussed in chapter 5, you should focus your plans for capital investment on the facilities that are essential to your hospital's initial operations. The architectural plans should be prepared in such a way as to ensure that the initial construction allows for future expansions at minimal cost.

Estimating Hard Costs

Hard costs are the most critical cost items that affect the financial viability of your project. They include the acquisition and preparation of land, the construction of buildings and infrastructure, and the purchase and installation of equipment, furniture, and fixtures.

LAND ACQUISITION AND PREPARATION

Your estimate of the costs for land acquisition and preparation and the timing of the payments will reflect the conditions of your agreement with the landowner. If you enter into a land purchase option agreement in order to secure the land for your hospital's future expansion, you may need to enter this as a land purchase cost in the project cost table, especially if the option agreement does not provide the possibility of cancellation. If the land purchase or leasing agreements are not finalized before the feasibility analysis is completed, as is often the case, you should reflect the best estimate in the initial projections and modify it as you firm up the agreement. It is also important to include various fees and taxes that will be associated with the acquisition and registration of the land when you estimate the land acquisition cost.

CONSTRUCTION

For the purpose of the feasibility analysis, you will estimate the cost of construction in consultation with your architect, your construction manager, and various construction companies. The construction of the hospital and auxiliary facilities is often done under a master contract at a fixed price. The magnitude of the construction cost will depend largely on the design of the hospital and the availability of locally produced construction materials of acceptable quality and price. The construction cost includes the cost of erecting the buildings and putting in any infrastructure that is needed, such as access roads, fencing, gas pipelines, a sewage system, a power generator, a waste disposal facility, and so on. Construction delays and cost overruns are among the most frequent problems for new projects. Thus you should consider, and factor in, the possibility of construction delays in the feasibility analysis. Chapter 9 discusses the tendering process for construction contracts and ways to cover the risks of construction delays.

EQUIPMENT PURCHASE AND INSTALLATION

Depending on the business and operating environment you are faced with, the selection of key medical equipment may be modified many times before it is finalized. You may need the help of a professional medical equipment planner (preferably an organization rather than an individual) to define your equipment needs, the selection criteria, and the selection process. In addition to contacting equipment suppliers, you should consult key physicians who will most likely practice at your hospital before making the final decision. Major medical equipment is discussed in chapter 8.

Professional assistance in medical equipment planning is available from independent advisory and research firms, which provide fee-based services including assessment of appropriate equipment choices for the services your hospital will provide, equipment management plans, price comparisons, and research information. When deciding whether to retain services of any of professional advisory service firm, you should obtain a clear understanding of the relationships between the advisory firm and any equipment manufacturers.

IT SYSTEMS

The cost of the IT systems, including the telecommunication systems, should include the cost of hardware and software, initial subscription fees, maintenance charges, and any consumable supplies needed to operate the systems properly.

Furniture, Fixtures, and Nonmedical Equipment

The cost of interior finishing, furniture, and fixtures can be high, depending on the choice of design and materials. Style, type and quality of material, and functionality in view of people's changing preferences need to be discussed with appropriate experts in this area before cost estimates are made.

Estimating Soft Costs

Project Development and Preopening

The distinction between the project development cost and the preopening cost is not always clear, as it is largely a matter of how to account for costs incurred up to the date of the hospital's opening. Generally, one can consider the project development cost to cover expenses incurred from the first days of developing the project concept up to the date of some critical event that marks the beginning of the project as a concrete reality, such as registration of the legal entity for the project. Expenditures incurred from that event up to the date of the facility's official opening would be considered the preopening cost. Some might consider the critical event to be the beginning of construction and start counting expenses from that point on (those expenses not directly connected with the construction) as preopening cost. The project development cost normally includes travel expenses, fees for lawyers and other consultants, fees or charges associated with market research and consumer surveys, and staff salaries. The preopening expenses include expenses related to establishment and registration of the project company, office rental charges, fees for lawyers and consultants, salaries of medical and administrative staff who will be hired before the opening of the hospital, training costs, office equipment and various supplies, marketing costs, financial charges incurred for the preopening period, and so forth.

The project development cost should be financed by seed (equity) capital, which is often provided by one or more persons who develop the project from its conceptual stage. The project's founding members who pay such expenses normally wish to have them accounted for as a part of the project's initial capital. In comparison, the preopening expenses are often partly funded by providers of loan as well as equity financing. Under the new international financial reporting system, all soft costs relating to the preopening period have to be expensed directly against the capital of the project company (the hospital's legal entity). This will have an important impact on the balance sheet of the project company during the initial years because it will reduce the equity base of the company by the amount of the development and preopening expenses. Many international financial institutions require certain minimum debt-to-equity ratios as a condition for their consideration to provide loan financing to any project. They also require that financial statements be prepared in accordance with the international financial reporting system. This means that you will need more equity capital to cover the soft costs in the early years of your project, in order to meet the ratio requirements, if you plan to obtain financing from international financial institutions. You should ask about the requirements and any possible flexibility in this regard when you discuss your project with potential lenders, especially international financial institutions.

Construction

The construction soft costs include fees paid to the architect and the construction manager, along with various taxes and other charges that are directly associated with the construction of the building. You will need the advice of an experienced lawyer to structure and negotiate appropriate terms and conditions for these professional services and the payment of fees. The architect's services will obviously be needed during the early stage of construction planning, but it is sometimes possible to negotiate payment of the architect's fees in installments that correspond to milestones in the project. The construction manager usually charges a monthly retainer fee plus a lump-sum amount that is payable upon completion of the construction.

Estimating Permanent Working Capital

One of the key reasons that projects fail early is an insufficient amount of permanent working capital. Working capital is needed to pay operating costs that are incurred before the payments for the hospital's services are collected in cash. If an analogy could be made, buildings and equipment are like the bones and muscles of a human body and working capital is like the blood that circulates through the body.

"Permanent" working capital is so called because once a business gets established and starts to grow the amount of working capital will continue to grow accordingly. Assuming that working capital is managed reasonably well, it is extremely unusual for the amount of working capital to decrease from the previous operating period in any normal business setting, unless there is a drastic change in the mode of operation. Once the hospital starts generating a sufficient extra cash flow (after paying monthly expenses and any debt service), its internally generated cash will be able to cover the additional working capital needed to support the growing volume of business. Until it can reach that point, however, the working capital has to be financed with externally sourced funds, either equity or loan.

Since the amount of working capital will not decrease once a business gets established and starts to grow, the amount of working capital needed during the first couple of years of your hospital's operation will become a "permanent" component of the presumably ever-growing working capital. Because of this characteristic, the permanent working capital needs to be financed with long-term financing and not with short-term loans or revolving credits. If the permanent working capital needed is financed with short-term financing, there will be a mismatch of funding that could cause unexpected financial difficulties in the first year or two of operation, a time when your hospital may have many other challenges to overcome.

Entrepreneurs and project developers and even consultants who conduct feasibility analyses often underestimate the need for permanent working capital. The main reasons for such underestimation are usually (a) lack of capital, (b) unrealistic expectations for initial success of the hospital's operations, and (c) insufficient analysis of the hospital's cash needs. When faced with an insufficient amount of capital, entrepreneurs are often tempted either to underestimate the working capital needs or to delay dealing with the issue until after the hospital's opening.

For a new project, the amount of working capital needed in the first 12 to 24 months after its opening has two components: (a) the amount of operating losses (costs that have been incurred for which the hospital has no one to charge), and (b) the amount of accounts receivable and inventories, plus other items such as temporary deposits and prepaid expenses (for example, insurance and taxes), less accounts payable. These two components both consist of operating costs and expenses for items such as salaries, medical supplies, and so on. Accounts receivable, for example, consist of the portion of the hospital's operating costs and expenses that are incurred in direct connection with the medical services for which the hospital can collect fees plus a profit margin. Depending on the credit quality of your patients, accounts receivable are expected to become cash inflow for your hospital within 15 to 30 days, though it often takes much longer in reality. If your hospital's revenues start rising quickly, say six months after its opening, the amount of working capital necessary will be close to item (b) noted above. For the hospital to be financially viable and profitable, the initial operating losses will have to be recovered from the hospital's future profits and net positive cash flows.

Once your hospital starts operation, you will need a clearly stated working capital management policy that is adhered to strictly. The most important working capital item is usually the accounts receivable. It is very important for the hospital to minimize its accounts receivable. To this end, you will need a policy statement that establishes payment conditions for all patients and defines who will qualify for delayed payments and under what conditions, who will monitor the status of receivables, and at what stage the hospital will stop providing services to clients who are delinquent on payments. In addition, the working capital management policy should include rules for management of cash, inventories, procurement of supplies, and accounts payable. Businesses usually try to collect account receivables sooner than the average period in which they pay accounts payable.

Estimating Financing Costs

Financing costs (including interest and fees) that will be incurred during the period leading up to the hospital's full operation need to be estimated and these estimates included in the project cost and financial plan. The estimates will depend on the structure of the financing arrangements. For example, estimating the interest will be simple if all the loans that you expect to obtain will carry fixed interest rates only. However, financing can be structured in a variety of ways, including income or revenue sharing, and each way requires certain assumptions for projection of financing costs. As a result, estimates of financing costs are often revised frequently in accordance with the progress being made in discussions with potential investors.

Contingencies

The two most important possibilities that require a good contingency plan are delays in completion of the physical facility (related to construction, equipment installation, setting up the IT system, connecting to communication channels, and so forth) and a slow buildup in operations that hampers revenue generation. There will be two elements to consider: what to do in case of delays in activity and who will bear the cost of delays. Defining specific performance thresholds for the construction contractor and holding the contractor responsible for the costs associated with delays will be one way of identifying risks and passing the cost of delay to another party.

Estimating how quickly the hospital will be able to build up its operations to a stable level is much more subjective and will depend on the quality of your market analysis, the effectiveness of your initial marketing activities, the on-time completion of construction and equipment installation within budget, the readiness of your medical and administrative staff with proper training, and of course smooth preparations for all logistical matters.

The approach often taken to contingency budgeting is to estimate 10–15 percent of construction cost and equipment cost (purchase and installation), assuming that these costs and working capital are prepared in a conservative and realistic manner. Depending on circumstances, you may need to budget as much as 20–25 percent of construction and equipment costs, but if the contingency budget is too high, it will cast doubt on the reasonableness of the base case budget.

The Financing Plan

It typically takes three to five years for a new hospital to firmly establish its reputation and start generating positive cash flow. For this reason, the total cost of establishing your hospital will need to be financed with long-term funds that do not place large payback burdens on the hospital soon after its opening. The financing plan has to consist of long-term funds only, such as equity, long-term loans, and quasi-equity (see chapter 5 for more discussions on these financing instruments). It is possible that you will be able to obtain short-term loans or revolving credit lines from local banks for your hospital's operation. However, at the beginning, the full financing plan should consist of long-term funds only, so that your hospital will not get into the financial difficulty discussed earlier in this chapter. Appendix J shows a sample table for a summary of project costs and financing plan.

In order to structure the financing plan, you will need to discuss with various potential financial partners the availability of financing and its conditions so that you can gain a reasonable sense of whether you will be able to obtain the financing necessary for your hospital. For the feasibility analysis, you will need indicative expressions of interest and willingness from your potential financial partners to finance your hospital and tentative terms and conditions of financing from each partner.

The pivotal element in your financing plan will be the amount of equity capital that can be mobilized. Grants that do not have any form of recovery or return conditions attached can be considered equity financing for the purpose of your financing plan. Providers of long-term loans or quasi-equity financing often require 35–50 percent of total project cost to be financed with equity for a new health care facility project, although the final requirement for the level of equity financing is determined after completion of financial projections based on the investors' own assessment of the project's viability and risks associated with it. In addition, many lenders require the availability of contingency funding over and above total project cost to cover cost overruns and greater-than-expected operating losses. Additional discussions of this topic are provided in chapter 5.

Preparing Financial Projections

At an early stage of your planning process, you will need to prepare a financial projection model (using Excel worksheets or a similar software program) to help you analyze the financial implications of each scenario in your project plan. The projection model is primarily a tool to assist your own analysis; sharing it with others is a secondary benefit. The model will reflect all of your thinking in terms of quantified units and can help you determine whether your plans have been thorough, reasonable, and realistic.

A sample format for selected sections of a financial projection model is provided in appendix K. Although a projection model is built using a computer software program, it should not be viewed as mechanical work and should not simply be delegated to a computer specialist or an accountant. Preparing a well-structured projection model cannot be done if the conceptual basis of your project and its key drivers are not well defined. The findings of your market research and analysis and the details of your plans will provide the basis for key assumptions that will drive the outcome of the projection model.

The person who builds the model should have a basic knowledge of accounting and financial matters so that he or she can help you analyze the logical interconnections between the projection assumptions, understand the financial and business implications of your plan, and define alternative assumptions. If you and your partners have the experience and the skills needed, you can build the projection model yourselves. If you do not, you can retain a consultant to prepare the model. However, keep in mind that you will need to use the financial projection model frequently later on—throughout the project's planning and development stages and even into an early stage of implementation—to update your plans and to test the financial impact of possible changes in your development and/or financing plans. Therefore, if someone who is not a member of the project team prepares the projection model, a member of your core project team should be trained to become fully knowledgeable about the model and should be able to modify key assumptions and the model itself if necessary.

Technical mistakes, such as data input mistakes in the projection model, are not uncommon. If you use a model that has mistakes in it, the consequences could be significant. Thus it is essential that the projection model and projections be reviewed and verified by someone other than the model builder. Try to keep the projection model from being structured in an overly elaborate and complicated manner.

It is impossible to overemphasize the importance of being conservative (that is, not overestimating revenues and underestimating costs and expenses) in determining key assumptions for the projection model. Some entrepreneurs worry that obtaining financing will be difficult if they do not show a bullish set of projections to potential financiers. In reality, overly optimistic numbers are likely to draw more skepticism than positive reactions.

As you develop the key parameters of the hospital's operations, you will be able to prepare a base case scenario for expected financial performance of the hospital. Once you have the base case scenario that demonstrates the viability of your project, you will need to prepare a round of sensitivity analyses for your projections.

The financial projections may be prepared in terms of constant currency units or nominal currency units. The difference between the two is the inclusion of inflation rates: nominal units include the inflation rate while constant units exclude inflation rates.

If you would like to project the hospital's financial performance in terms of nominal currency value, you would consider the likely inflation rate for each of the projection periods and determine each key monetary assumption in nominal value. When doing so, you should consider that some items may increase at less than the average inflation rate while others may increase faster than the average inflation rate. If your hospital will be built in a region that may have an inflationary pattern different from the national average, regional differences should be taken into consideration.

If you elect to prepare the projections in constant currency terms, you will consider the prices and costs in "real" terms without adding the effect of inflation. When you do so, you need to make sure to include the "real" increase or decrease in the prices and costs. If you expect that the hospital will not be able to pass the full extent of the inflation rate on to its patients by way of price increases, the prices of the hospital's services would show a decreasing pattern, assuming that creeping inflation is expected, over the projection period under the constant currency unit model.

Estimating Revenues and Operating Costs and Expenses

REVENUES

As in any other business, the level of revenues of a hospital is the most important determinant of its financial success. Provided that the pricing is right and cash collection is not a problem, rising revenues will be the strongest indicator of the hospital's successful operations. Optimistic estimation of revenues, especially for the first two to three years of the project's operation, is one of the most common and serious mistakes in planning for any project. It should be strenuously avoided.

Some entrepreneurs project the hospital's revenues in a simplistic way, such as by estimating revenues for each department (for example, pediatrics, internal medicine) on the basis of either informed intuition or the opinions of knowledgeable physicians. With regard to the latter, there may be considerable differences in nature and scope between the practices of advising physicians and your hospital's operations. One or two seemingly small differences in the operational environment can cause considerable differences in revenues. Some entrepreneurs also obtain data on the amount of revenues generated by existing hospitals—although such data are almost always limited—and make adjustments for their own projects. However, unless you have a good understanding of the differences in the operational settings of the hospitals that are used as comparators, your estimations may be fundamentally flawed. Still others simply project total revenues based on an average revenue per patient, irrespective of specific intervention.

Going about this task in a methodical, systematic way does not guarantee that the estimations will match reality. However, such a projection of revenues helps you in your capital investment decisions, such as those regarding medical equipment (the most frequent source of overspending), auxiliary facilities, or patient amenities. For example, if you wanted to buy a magnetic resonance imaging (MRI) machine—often cited as necessary to establish a new hospital's reputation and attract patients—you might find out that you will probably not be able to generate enough cash to pay for the machine and still make the necessary profit margin on that investment.

The best way to quantify the projected levels of services will differ for each functional department (for example, operating room, oncology department) and for each category of procedures. Once you have determined the basis for quantifying the activity level of each department or category of procedures, you will need to estimate the average revenue per procedure or per patient. When you make these estimates, all revenue items that could be generated in relation to each procedure or patient should be identified and aggregated, rather than simply using the price for each procedure.

When making decisions on pricing and preparing financial projections, you may look into the possibility of charging and receiving fees in hard currencies, if local regulations allow it. In some countries and markets, it may be possible to quote prices in hard currency terms but receive payments in local currency only. If the prices can be quoted in hard currency, your hospital may be able to protect its revenue base in terms of local currency by transferring the currency devaluation risk to patients through pricing adjustments. If a substantial portion of the hospital's revenues can be generated in foreign currency, you will need to estimate it separately and reflect the impact of hard currency earnings in the projection model.

OPERATING COSTS AND EXPENSES

Usually the most important cash items in this category are staff salaries, supplies (pharmaceutical, medical, and other), and utilities. Depreciation of the book value of buildings and equipment will also be a major cost item in the hospital's income statement, but it will be an accounting cost item rather than a cash item. If your hospital will have other activities that can add significant value to its operations and its cash generation, your cost structure will also reflect such items.

Determining key drivers of cost and expense items is straightforward for some items but not for others. For example, estimation of staff salaries obviously will be based on the number of staff that will be on duty at different times. Once you decide on the average salaries, taxes, and benefits per person, it will be a relatively simple exercise to estimate the employee-related costs. However, even in this case you will need to validate the appropriateness of the assumptions by cross-checking on the manpower needs in light of the expected level of activity of each profit center and cost center. In projecting operating costs and expenses, you will need to consider the effect of efficiency gains that could be realized after one or two years of your hospital's operations.

The purchase cost of pharmaceutical products will depend on the type of purchasing terms and payments that can be arranged. The estimated pharmaceutical costs should include allowances for spoilage and loss of items due to expiration dates, poor storage conditions, and other reasons.

Once the hospital starts operations, staff training will need to continue at a substantial level during the first 12 to 24 months. This will be in addition to the training costs that are incurred as a part of the preopening preparations. Marketing and sales promotion costs will need to reflect your marketing and sales strategy. In many cases, the marketing and sales budget is set at a certain percentage of net revenues.

CAPITAL EXPENDITURES

After the first couple of years, you will need to start upgrading and/or replacing equipment as items wear out or become obsolete. As the hospital's operation starts to grow, more equipment and aspects of the IT systems will need to be maintained and/or replaced. You must budget for these capital expenditure items and reflect them in the financial projections.

Estimating Cash Flows

The cash flow generated from operations, after all operating costs and expenses have been paid off, is used for two main purposes: to reinvest in the business and to pay back the capital that was invested in the project. The latter entails debt service (repayment of principal plus interest) as well as payment of dividends and other forms of profit sharing. The pro forma cash flow statement needs to show that there will be a sufficient amount of "free" cash flow, that is, cash that will be available for servicing debt and paying dividends. Free cash flow means the amount of cash obtained from operations after all operating expenses have been paid off, minus the amount of additional working capital needed during the relevant operating period, and minus the amount of capital expenditures needed to keep up with normal operations (excluding large special capital expenditures such as expansion cost, which has to be financed with external financing). Lenders usually require that the free cash flow be at least 20–30 percent more than the amount of debt service (loan repayment and interests) for each projection period.

If your projections show negative or inadequate free cash flow for any given year or projection period, simply assuming that a short-term loan will solve the problem is probably not the best way to manage. Rather, you should identify the causes of the cash shortfall and make the necessary changes in your project and total project costs, as well as estimated operating costs, to address the problem at the beginning.

Estimating Financial Viability

INDICATORS OF FINANCIAL VIABILITY

The most frequently used indicators of financial viability include gross operating margin, operating margin, debt-to-equity ratio, debt service ratio, financial rate of return of the project, and financial return on equity. The internal rate of return (IRR) of the project is calculated based on the net present value of all free cash flows over the projection period, plus a residual value of the business's assets at the end of the projection period, minus net present value of total project cost. The objective of testing the IRR on total project cost is to see whether or not investing the amount of total capital needed for your project would be an efficient use of capital. The benchmark IRR on total project cost differs depending on the perspectives of each investor or lender, but 15 percent or higher in real terms is commonly regarded as a minimum required rate. Return on equity investment is calculated net of scheduled debt service (payment of interests and repayment of principal). Equity investors in general would tend to require a higher rate of return on their investments in the project.

If the financial projection results show weak viability after you have verified the model and the assumptions, you will need to revisit the business strategy and capital cost structure.

A series of "what if" scenarios are prepared to test the resilience of the project's financial viability. Having completed the base case scenario projections, you will need to identify the major risk areas and modify the relevant assumptions negatively to see how the hospital's financial results will differ from the base case scenario.

The sensitivity test could be carried out, for example, by lowering the amount of estimated revenues, especially for the first two years, by 25–40 percent. This can be achieved by reducing either the estimated quantity of services or the prices of services, or both. Here again, the important point is that the sensitivity analysis must be carried out based on clearly understandable rationales so that the analysis will be beneficial to you. The objective is to see how far the hospital can withstand events that could have negative impacts on its revenues and cash flow. If modifying one or more key assumptions has the potential to cause serious financial downturns for the hospital, you will need to revisit the operational plans to make modifications that would render the hospital less vulnerable to particular risks.

Will Your Hospital Be Viable?

At the end of the feasibility analysis, you should be able to ascertain the following in order to know whether or not your project's viability can be demonstrated:

- The hospital can be built without major problems and within the overall budget and time frame.
- The hospital can operate without serious worry of disruption (for example, power shortages, lack of necessary personnel, floods, social unrest, nearby construction or serious pollution).
- The hospital can generate enough cash to pay for all its operating expenses, increases in working capital, and capital expenditures required for proper upkeep of its facilities; service its debts; and pay dividends and other obligations associated with share capital.

- The base case financial projections are realistic and reasonable enough to allow a high level of confidence that the estimated cash flows can be generated as expected.
- The hospital can operate without serious concern about environmental or health hazards and/or worker safety issues.
- A sufficient amount of funds can be sourced in time and on terms and conditions that the hospital's cash flow can afford.

A Note on the Business Plan

The business plan is an evolving document that will reflect the status of the project, and therefore it is common to revise it as the project develops. At the beginning, the business plan will be a relatively short document that sets forth initial ideas for the project and potential highlights. As details of the project are developed, more information will be added. The results of the prefeasibility analysis and, later on, of each iteration of the feasibility analysis will have a significant impact on the business plan.

As discussed in chapter 7, by the time the hospital's design development documents are prepared, the architectural plans for the hospital will be substantially determined, allowing finalization of the total project cost. At this stage, the feasibility analysis will be finalized and so will the business plan. The final business plan will include copies of the conceptual sketches for the hospital and may even include copies of certain sections of the schematic design drawings, as well as the results of the finalized base case financial projections. Therefore, it is possible that you may prepare and submit to banks and other potential partners several versions of the business plan, each of which will demonstrate the advancing status of the project.

5

Obtaining Financing

Keeping Your Fuel Tank Filled

One of the most common reasons given for failure of an investment project is that the project "ran out of money." The simple fact is that projects do not just run out of money. Rather, it is typically a combination of poor financial planning and bad luck. If you fail to back up your project by raising enough cash, you may lose your dreams and all your hard work may be wasted.

Historically, private health care facilities have generally not been active participants in financial markets. Hospitals, like many other health care facilities, are often thought to be social service providers first and businesses second, if at all. The idea that a health care facility should aim to be profitable has yet to be fully embraced in many countries. Therefore, obtaining financing for a private hospital remains a very challenging undertaking.

In many developing countries, private health care services have mostly been small operations, often owned and managed by individual practitioners. Small private clinics that develop into hospitals usually do so after a decade or so of successful operations. Such a pattern of development usually does not require large amounts of external financing, as such clinics can usually rely on their own cash generation to build hospitals. Owners of small and medium-size private hospitals—who often are also practitioners at the facilities—are usually not familiar with the process of obtaining external financing, and they tend to be wary of inviting outsiders (especially nonmedical persons) into their businesses.

At the same time, there are large private hospitals that have been operating successfully in many middle-income countries. Most of them were established by local business groups driven by the desire to provide social services as part of their corporate social responsibility, often coupled with the desire to take advantage of tax benefits. Such hospitals usually rely on funds from the business group's own cash generation or the estate of the entrepreneur who started the business group, and not on external financing such as bank loans.

Such a pattern of development of private hospitals means that commercial banks in general have not often been asked to provide loans to private hospitals. Nor have they reached out to private hospitals in search of lending opportunities, as the banks often prefer to pursue large infrastructure or industry projects. As a result, relatively few banking sector professionals are experienced in analyzing the business viability of private hospitals. In some countries, local laws prevent physical assets of private health care facilities from being mortgaged, adding more constraint to lending considerations by commercial banks. Even if the assets can be mortgaged, banks might feel that they may not be able to enforce their mortgage rights when necessary because such an action might disrupt the hospital's operations.

There are exceptional cases, such as Bumrungrad Hospital in Bangkok, Thailand, and the Apollo Hospital Group in India, which reportedly have successfully obtained external financing from international financial institutions. On the lending side, a few multilateral financial institutions such as International Finance Corporation have taken the initiative to actively seek opportunities to support viable private health care facilities in developing countries in recent years. These types of institutions are also exploring innovative financing mechanisms—for example, financing for public-private partnership programs—to provide broader support to the development of private health care in developing countries.

Keys to Success in Obtaining Financing

What, then, will make it possible to successfully raise the funds needed for your hospital? It will depend, of course, on many aspects of the economic and business environment and capital markets in the country where your hospital will be located. Nonetheless, certain criteria are generally applicable.

First and foremost, your concept has to be sensible and realistic. Second, investors will want to know that the project's sponsors have sufficient experience and knowledge about the health care industry and what it takes to successfully establish a new hospital. The amount of equity financing that can be provided by the sponsors will also be seen as indicating their seriousness about the project and their capability to see it through.

The third important element that investors will look at is the track record and quality of the senior management team that will operate the hospital after its construction, as well as the project management team that will be responsible for the planning and implementation of the project's plan.

Also important is a sound financial plan that includes a sufficient level of equity financing and a credible plan for obtaining the target amount of equity. In addition, your plan has to demonstrate, in a logical way, your project's technical, operational, and financial viability in the context of the overall economic and business environment in the country and locality where your hospital will be established. All of the above-noted elements and other details have to be explained well in a business plan (see appendix L).

If you are not familiar with the concepts and jargon related to banking and financing, it would be a good idea to gain basic knowledge and advice at an early stage of your planning. For example, you could consult a professor of finance at a university near you. You might need to pay consulting fees, but it will be worth the money and time invested. If you feel uncomfortable dealing directly with banks and other financing sources, you may wish to consider retaining a financial consultant.

Finally, do not expect that investors will provide funding to support your project because it is a great project from the social service point of view. Similarly, you cannot assume that funds will be disbursed just because agreements have been signed. There are several steps you must go through before you can actually receive the money.

Managing Cash Flows and Recordkeeping

Throughout the process of establishing your hospital, the most critical challenge will be matching cash inflow with cash outflow. As you proceed with further planning of your hospital, you must have daily, weekly, and monthly cash flow (cash in and out) worksheets in detail. These should be consistent with the base case financial projections, so far as possible, from the early stages of your project's planning and development.

The actual handling of cash should always be done through bank accounts, and handling of cash should be minimized for better recordkeeping. Often an entrepreneur starts spending her own money early on for travel, consultation with lawyers, and so forth, without proper recording. After a certain time, the amount of funds spent becomes considerable, but without proper documentary evidence the entrepreneur finds it difficult to prove that she has spent her own funds. All invoices and receipts for expenditures incurred and paid should be filed in a well-organized manner. Another aspect often overlooked by entrepreneurs is keeping daily records of events, plans made, meetings held, promises made (both by you and to you), and commitments kept.

It would be very helpful if you could hire, at an early stage of your planning, one or more administrative staffers who have good knowledge of accounting and finance. If it is costly or impractical to hire someone directly, you could consider obtaining the assistance of an accounting firm to provide the bank account management, recordkeeping, and financial reporting services for monthly fees of fixed amounts.

Spending versus Paying

The difference between spending (that is, incurring legal and moral obligation to pay) and actually making cash payments is an important distinction that many people fail to recognize. During the project planning, construction, and preopening stages, controlling spending is much more important to good cash management than delaying cash payments. During these stages, deferred payments must be limited to the absolute minimum possible so that one can avoid failing to complete the project and ending up with a pile of unpaid invoices and unmet promises to pay.

How to Look for Financing

When do you need to start looking for funds? The answer is at the same time that you first start thinking about your project. Because the scope and key elements of your project can be firmed up realistically only when you have a high degree of certainty about financing, you will need to start discussions with your potential financial partners early on and look for ways to match their requirements with the needs of your project as you develop its details.

The first step is to obtain as much information as possible about various types and sources of funds that might be available for your project. These include, among others:

- Government ministries and agencies
- Government-owned or government-controlled banks and nonbank financial institutions such as guarantee agencies
- Bilateral aid agencies such as the United States Agency for International Development (USAID)
- Domestic and foreign private commercial banks
- Private nonbank financial institutions such as leasing companies
- International development finance institutions
- Private equity funds
- Equipment suppliers
- Philanthropic foundations
- Nongovernmental organizations (NGOs)
- Auditors and financial consultants
- Wealthy individuals

As you visit the potential financiers, be sure to ask as many questions as possible about various regulations, the organization's objectives, their operating policies, their organizational structures, financing programs (debt or equity, or both), criteria for financing decisions, conditions for financing, the application process, the decision-making processes, paperwork needed, the critical milestones, and the average amount of time needed for final approval. Appendix M provides some information on potential sources of financing.

Your knowledge about the possible sources of funds, the types of funds (such as grants, equity investments, and long-term loans), and the conditions attached to funds will help determine how you shape your project and how you present it to potential investors. If you know which aspects of your project would make it easier to qualify or meet the preferences and/or requirements of various funding sources, you will be able to develop your project in a way that is consistent with your vision and objectives while also meeting the needs and objectives of your potential financial partners.

More than any other aspect of your project, the process of seeking funding will test your patience and your capacity to absorb the ups and downs associated with a large venture. You cannot count on funding until you have written commitments. Although such commitments are sometimes first provided in preliminary and nonbinding form, it is important to obtain the potential investors' positions in writing as you proceed with each step.

Whom to Approach First

The first group of potential financial partners should be providers of grants and equity financing. This is because the amount and structure of equity financing is the most critical element in mobilizing debt financing. Banks usually will not consider a project seriously unless there is a high level of certainty about the amount and conditions of equity financing available for the project. Grants, if they can be obtained, will at best constitute a small portion of your project's financing plan. In most developing countries, grants generally are not easily available from domestic sources. Instead, they tend to be available from international bilateral or multilateral donors, international NGOs, and private philanthropic foundations that operate internationally. Equity financing is also usually difficult to obtain, especially from investors who seek commercial rates of return on their investments.

The most typical first source of equity financing is the partners who share your vision and goals. The most typical situation is that the partners put together as much money as possible for initial equity financing and then try to leverage these funds by expanding the search to colleagues, friends, family members, banks, or wealthy individuals who might be willing to support the project.

Hospitals Owned and Managed by Physicians

Many private hospitals have been successfully established by a large group of physicians who provided equity financing and became shareholders. In most cases, the physicians also manage the hospital by electing a management team from among their peer shareholders. Most such hospitals operate in the country where the physician-shareholders are located.

The larger the number of physicians who are targeted to become equity investors in a private hospital, the more complex and challenging will be the process of obtaining the needed financing. If you are going to design your hospital to be physician-owned and physician managed, you will need to think through key matters at a relatively early stage of your fundraising efforts. This means asking the following questions, among others:

- What is the theme that will appeal to target physicians?
- What will be offered as the primary reason for investing in the hospital? Will it be priority rights to use the facilities for the physicians' own patients, the right to purchase a space at the hospital's complex, an opportunity to do social good, a promise of high financial returns, or some combination of the above?
- What other special rights, if any, could you offer to the physician-shareholders and at what stage of the hospital's development could they be offered?
- What will be the responsibilities, if any, of the physician-shareholders in addition to providing equity financing? In other words, will the physicians be equity investors only, or will they also work at the hospital?
- If the physicians will work at the hospital while being shareholders in the business, will they be subject to same work and other performance requirements as physicians (and members of the hospital's management team) who are not shareholders?
- How will the physician-shareholders participate in the hospital's management? If they are allowed to join the management team, what kind of system will be put in place to handle problems that could arise from a clash of egos and personalities?
- What decision-making process and operating policies will be put in place to ensure that the hospital will benefit from hiring competent and experienced noninvestor physicians and/or nonphysician managers, including the procedures for firing and replacing managers?
- How will the compensation packages for members of the management team be determined, especially if most members of the management team are going to be physician-shareholders?

- What will be the responsibilities of the physician-shareholders if additional funds are needed, either to complete the construction of the hospital or to finance working capital shortfalls after the hospital has started operations?
- How can the physician-shareholders sell their shares if they wish to sell? Can they sell the shares before the hospital is completed, or should they be required to keep the shares and not sell for a fixed number of years? Should they be required to offer their shares to other physicians before offering them to outsiders?

The fundraising documents that will be necessary if you decide to raise financing from a large number of physicians should include, among others, a shareholders' agreement and/or articles of incorporation, which should cover most of the questions noted above.

Documenting Promises from Both Sides

Whether you turn to professional colleagues, friends, or family members for the first round of financing, it is necessary to document in writing any arrangements you make with them. Requiring documentation when dealing with close associates is not common, and in many cultures may even be thought of as a sign of lack of trust. However, putting things in writing not only can save the time that might be spent on unnecessary arguments in the future, but can also help protect your friendships, professional relationships, and family ties from the potentially corrosive effects of money disputes.

Types of Financing

Even though it is challenging to raise funds for health care facilities, today's sophisticated financial markets offer various types of financing to projects that demonstrate technical, operational, and financial viability. There are two broad categories of funds: those that carry a contractual obligation to repay and those that do not. Obviously, the more nonrepayable financing you can obtain, the better it will be for your project's financial viability.

Funds that do not carry legal repayment obligations include grants, equity, and certain types of quasi-equity financing such as nonredeemable preferred shares. Loans are the most typical type of financing with the obligation to repay. The various ways in which different types of financing can be structured are discussed in the following section.

Regardless of the type of financing, any and all external funds will come at a price. In the case of loans, the price comes in the form of fees, interest charges, and security packages (for example, guarantees and mortgage rights over assets). In the case of equity, it comes in the form of a share of profits and ownership rights. In the case of grants, the grantee's obligation is to ensure that the money is spent as promised.

Local Currency versus Foreign Currency Financing

When you consider whether to seek loans in local or foreign currency, the latter may appear more attractive because of the lower interest rate (provided that you can qualify for a foreign currency loan). However, you will need to weigh other elements in addition to the interest rate before making a decision on the mix of loans in different currencies. This is important because a hospital's revenues are typically generated in local currency; thus, when a hospital takes out a foreign currency loan, it will assume the risk of currency mismatch in its cash flows.

The first aspect to consider is the project's need for hard currency, both for costs related to the physical completion of the hospital and for ongoing operation after the opening. You should draw up a list of anticipated payments, with their expected timing, for imported medical equipment and supplies, IT software purchases, any particular construction material that you would need to import (if the construction manager cannot do so), salaries of foreign personnel, and other such expenses. Other ongoing hard currency needs would include fees associated with maintenance and upgrading of medical equipment and the IT system.

The second element to consider is the likelihood of devaluation of the local currency (box 5.1). A sudden and severe devaluation of local currency will cause a steep increase in the amount of local currency needed to pay back a foreign currency loan in a very short period of time. Because it will be nearly impossible for the hospital to pass this increase fully to its patients in the form of higher charges, the hospital will have to quickly find large sums of local currency to make the loan repayment and interest payment. In such a situation, the all-in cost of a foreign currency loan will become much higher than initially expected, and the foreign currency loan could thus become more expensive than a local currency loan over time.

It is imperative that you obtain sufficient information about the exchange rate risk and include this risk in your assessment of the overall cost of financing involving local and foreign currencies. You should develop several different scenarios reflecting possible changes in exchange rates at different times. These scenarios should take into account how the devaluation of the local currency would affect other cost items and in what time frame. You can then test the

Box 5.1 Dealing with Foreign Exchange Risk

In 1999 the Brazilian government, in an effort to boost exports and achieve a positive trade balance, decided to devaluate the *real* by more than 100 percent. Many hospitals that had debt denominated in foreign currency were exposed and at risk. Some of these hospitals lost their favorable financial positions, and a few even went bankrupt. The HMSL Group in São Paulo, however, had made a prudent decision that later proved to be beneficial to the group. After analyzing global market liquidity, macroeconomic conditions in Brazil, and their own hospital's debt and equity ratios, the financial management team of HMSL decided to hedge half of its foreign currency debt in U.S. dollars. The decision in favor of dollars was based on an assessment, later confirmed, that the euro was undervalued. This example shows that financial managers must take into account not only interest rates but also potential foreign exchange risks when evaluating financing options.

overall impact of such scenarios on your prices and costs, and on your hospital's financial viability and cash flow, before making a final decision about currency. If you decide to take out foreign currency loans, you should look into the possibility of mitigating the foreign currency risk through currency swaps or hedging if there is a sufficiently developed market for such products in the country where your hospital will operate.

Choosing a Mix of Funds

Questions about how much financing can be raised in the form of equity, debt, leasing, quasi-equity (mezzanine) financing, and grants are interrelated. In other words, the decisions made by equity investors will affect the decisions of lenders and vice versa, especially because such decisions are made in an iterative way. Each potential investor will want to know how firm the commitments of other investors are before making their own commitments. The commitment that provides the most critical starting point is that of equity financing. Banks usually will not take your project seriously unless you can demonstrate that you have a firm commitment, or a credible preliminary commitment, of significant equity financing from credible investors.

As discussed in chapter 4, the level of equity financing that most lenders will require for a new hospital project is in the range of 33 to 50 percent of total financing needed (including the estimated permanent working capital discussed in chapter 4). Depending on the country and specifics of a project, the percentage of loan financing that banks might be willing to consider could be as low as 50 percent. The percentages referred to above are provided as a general point of reference and are not meant to suggest that these numbers are used as a standard rule by all lending institutions.

Structure of Financing

When discussions with your potential financial partners reach a certain level of seriousness, you will need to examine how each component of the financing plan can be structured. This means determining the types of financing instruments that will be used for each cost item and the kinds of terms and conditions each financing instrument could contain.

Grants

Grants are provided by governments, religious organizations, international organizations, public and private philanthropic foundations, large corporations, and individuals. In some countries, South Africa for example, corporations are required by law to spend a certain portion of their annual profits for social purposes. The grant providers give grants to satisfy their own predetermined objectives and, in most cases, without any expectation of getting the money back.

Most grant givers have different "facilities" of funds that are set aside for specific types of activities to fulfill specific purposes. You need to understand fully the objectives, the modes of operation, the requirements to qualify for funding, and other conditions attached to each grant facility before approaching the grant provider. In addition, you may consider whether or not your project's design and/or activities could be tailored, at an early stage, to satisfy conditions set by the grant provider(s) to the extent possible without having to alter your vision.

Grants usually support programs and/or activities and tend to finance soft costs, such as staff salaries and consultant fees. Grants are rarely provided for hard costs such as construction or equipment, although some private philanthropic foundations provide funds to build community health care centers, immunization centers, and the like, and then donate them to the communities or organizations upon completion. Because grants usually finance activities or programs, the grant providers usually require completion reports, and possibly proof of payment as well, to confirm that the money has been spent in keeping with the grant objectives.

With the increasing awareness that health care is a critical foundation for economic and social development, some philanthropic foundations and NGOs are becoming more willing to consider providing grants as seed capital—that is, equity—for private health care facilities in developing countries.

Some countries have a fairly large diaspora, with many of their nationals well established professionally and financially in foreign countries. These individuals may be ready to consider financing support for a new hospital project through either grants or equity investments. If your research leads you to tap into the diaspora community, be sure to allocate sufficient time and effort for planning and managing the process of marketing your project and fundraising. You may consider obtaining the services of a professional fundraising management company that will provide the necessary services for a fee.

Equity Financing

Typically, equity financing is provided in the form of subscription to a company's common shares. As such, it does not carry any legal obligation to pay back the funds. However, an equity financing can be structured in a variety of ways, including some that contain a condition to return the original capital investment in accordance with a predetermined schedule or method.

COMMON SHARES

The most typical and straightforward way to structure an equity financing is through issuance of common shares in the project company and/or in a holding company that owns the project company. The project company is normally the legal entity that owns the hospital, although there are exceptions to this as some countries do not allow direct ownership of social service facilities such as hospitals. In most cases, however, the project company is also the borrower of loans to be used for the hospital. Common shares represent a piece of the ownership of the company and the entitlement to a share of profits that will be made by the company in the future. As such, most common shares are issued with voting rights to key decisions that affect the company's operations and its future, but without any stated obligation for the company to redeem (that is, pay back) the shares.

By definition, shareholders of a limited liability company are responsible for the financial consequences of the company only up to the extent of the equity investment they have made. Therefore, shareholders lose their investments if the company fails, but they are normally not responsible for other liabilities of the company. In exchange for the limited liability and the entitlement to the company's future earnings, holders of common shares are the last to be compensated if the company is liquidated either voluntarily or involuntarily.

Matters concerning the type, number, and terms and conditions of shares that can be issued by a limited liability company are determined by the company's articles of association, which in turn have to comply with the relevant laws and regulations of the country where the company would be incorporated. The articles of association normally define the decisions that would require the approval of all shareholders, the total number of shares authorized to be issued, and the number of shares that can be actually issued (sold) at a given time, as well as many other important matters such as the structure of the board of directors.

In addition to common voting shares, equity financing can be structured in a variety of ways, all of which are essentially variations of common shares. The variations can take the form of preferential treatments relating to payment of dividends, redemption rights, recovery of investment at the time of liquidation, and conversion rights. Equity financing arrangements that involve such variations are generally referred to as equity-type quasi-equity financing.[9]

PREFERRED SHARES

Preferential treatments often include payment of dividends at a predetermined rate, redemption of shares, recovery of capital at the time of the company's liquidation, and other special conditions that can be tailored to the specific requirements of the equity investor.

When a company issues a stock of preferred shares with special rights to dividend payments, the company creates for itself an obligation to pay dividends in accordance with the terms and conditions that are specified in relevant agreements. Preferred dividend payments can be determined based on the company's net income, operating income, or revenues, either quarterly, biannually, or annually. More discussion on preferred shares is provided in appendix N.

EXIT MECHANISMS FOR EQUITY INVESTMENTS

Some equity investors may wish to have a way to exit and recover from the investment. The most typical way to exit from an equity investment is through exercise of a put option. A put option agreement specifies terms and conditions under which the holder of the put rights would be able to demand that the put obligor buy back the shares that are subject to the put agreement. The put obligor could be other shareholders, the company, or in rare cases, a third party.

From the perspectives of an issuer of preferred shares, there has to be sufficient compensation for providing an investor with various preferential treatments. The compensation could be in the form of a premium on the price of shares and/or subscription of the shares by a date prior to the issuance of common shares. Another common "price" charged for various preferential treatments is the lack of voting rights. In other words, you might consider agreeing to pay mandatory dividends or to buy back the shares in exchange for excluding the

---

9.   Quasi-equity financing is also commonly called mezzanine financing, as it combines many features of loans and common shares.

investor from having a say in how the hospital would be run. Conversely, a veto right can be used as an incentive to a particular investor who is willing to provide equity financing in exchange for having control over certain aspects of the hospital's operation. When carefully considered and structured, a veto right could provide you and your partners with a valuable way to mobilize equity financing without incurring extra financing cost. Shares with special rights are often issued with the condition that such shares cannot be sold to other parties without written consent of the company and/or other shareholders.

Any of the variations noted above would have financial consequences and could affect the decisions of lenders and other equity investors. For example, mandatory dividend payments and redemption schedules would have the same effect as a typical debt service and could therefore cause a reduction in the amount of loan you would be able to obtain. Lenders and other potential equity investors may be reluctant to participate in the project if you have already agreed to give too many incentives to a particular investor. Therefore, you will need to carefully consider, with appropriate legal advice, using any of the features discussed above and ensure that the structure of any particular financing arrangement would not affect negatively the structure and timing of the remainder of the financing needed.

Debt Financing

Today's financial markets offer a wide variety of financing mechanisms that are tailored to meet the various needs of different individuals and corporations. You might consider the following financing options, which are generally available from the banking sector in many countries: (a) short-term credit facilities such as revolving credit lines that are often unsecured, (b) term loans of medium- and long-term maturity, and (c) debt-type quasi-equity financing of medium- and long-term maturity. The main features of a typical term loan and a debt-type quasi-equity financing instrument are often combined to structure a financing package that is suitable for the project and acceptable to lenders and the borrower. Banks generally do not provide unsecured short-term credit facilities to a start-up company, so such an arrangement would probably be available only after the hospital has been completed and has established an acceptable track record of revenues and cash flow generation. For the purposes of meeting your financing needs to construct and establish the hospital, either a typical term loan or a debt-type quasi-equity financing instrument or a combination of both would be more appropriate.

INTEREST RATES

The key variables that affect the structure of debt and debt-type quasi-equity financing instruments include the interest rates, the conditions of repayment of the loan principal, and the security package. Many first-time project developers start their discussions with banks by asking about interest rates, thinking that the interest is the most important aspect of a loan. But the interest rate alone does not determine the full cost of a loan. It is only one of several key components of a debt financing package, albeit an important one. When visiting a bank, you should first ask what kind of financing instruments the bank might be able to offer for a project such as yours, as there are many different ways in which debt financing can be designed.

The interest rate can be set as either a fixed rate or a variable rate. A variable interest rate has two components: an index rate and a spread. The index rate most often used by international banks is three- or six-month LIBOR (London interbank offered rate), or interest rates on certain bonds issued by central governments. The spread is negotiated in consideration of various risk factors, including the project's viability and prospects, quality of the management team, maturity of the loan, repayment conditions, foreign exchange risks, quality of the security package, and other potential issues and risks. The spread can be structured to vary at a certain interval, depending on the project's physical completion (for example, the spread could decrease after the project has been fully completed on time and on budget), its operational and financial performance, the start of repayment of the principal, or other milestone events. Some lenders might offer an opportunity to switch, for a fee, from fixed to variable or vice versa during the life of the loan, so that borrowers can benefit from declining interest rate trends without having to refinance the entire amount of the outstanding loan.

REPAYMENT CONDITIONS

The most typical repayment schedule calls for installment payments of equal amounts at set intervals, usually twice a year, over a number of years. Repayments usually start after the end of a grace period during which only interest payments are made. The repayment amounts do not always have to be equal amounts, but can vary according to the project's needs and negotiations with the lender, from year to year or every two or three years. In view of the time needed for a new hospital to build up its revenues, the repayments in the first couple of years, after the grace period has ended, could start as relatively small amounts; the amounts would then increase in later years as the hospital's operations are established and its cash flows improve. In some cases, lenders might be willing to consider a bullet repayment, meaning that the loan principal would become payable in one lump sum at the end of the loan maturity period, say, seven or eight years after the financing is provided. The grace period and repayment schedules determine the effective maturity of a loan. Lenders consider that the longer the maturity of a loan, the riskier it will be. The lender would therefore charge a higher interest rate for loans with longer effective maturities to compensate for the higher risk.

SECURITY REQUIREMENTS

When structuring a debt financing package, lenders normally prefer a full recourse financing under which they would have a sure way to get their loans and interest back. This is often achieved by having an unconditional guarantee that another party will repay the loan and all of the interest that would accumulate on the loan if the borrower fails to do so. Such a guarantee would be in the form of either a letter of credit or a letter of guarantee issued by a financially strong financial institution.

For projects for which such guarantees cannot be provided, a limited-recourse financing package can be structured. The idea is to provide the lender with a sufficient level of comfort that it will recover at least a substantial portion of its capital. Such a package usually includes a mixture of mortgage rights over the borrower's fixed assets, as well as certain current assets if local law allows it, and other forms of security. The latter could include a pledge of shares in the borrower company, which could provide the lenders with an additional channel to recover their investment. A debt financing package is called project financing when it is based on a structure whereby the lenders rely mainly on a project's expected cash flow and its assets, and not on a third party, to obtain the interest and repayment of the loan. In reality, project financing packages often include some form of guarantees as well as security over the project's assets.

COVENANTS AND EVENTS OF DEFAULT

In addition to the above, lenders usually attach to loans various nonfinancial conditions called covenants. Covenants specify certain actions that the borrower must either take (positive covenants) or avoid (negative covenants). Typical positive covenants include reporting requirements, insurance coverage, and measures related to good governance, while the most common negative covenants involve prohibition of increasing indebtedness, prohibition of paying dividends, and so forth. Another important nonfinancial matter included in loan financing agreements is the definition of events of default. The events of default provision usually specifies a variety of situations that would give the lender a right to call that the borrower is in default, even when the loan is being serviced on time.

DEBT-TYPE QUASI-EQUITY FINANCING

Debt-type quasi-equity financing instruments combine the elements of typical loans noted above with additional features that provide lenders with potentially higher returns in exchange for taking higher risks than the risks associated with a typical term loan. Some lenders might consider taking higher risks in the form of longer grace periods, lower interest rates, longer repayment periods, subordinated rights, or a weaker security package than what they would normally require. Lenders will seek to be compensated for such higher risks by requiring higher interest rates in later years, a special up-front fee, a portion of the hospital's income or revenues in addition to the coupon interest rate, call option for a lump-sum payment after a certain period (that is, forced prepayment), conversion rights from loan into equity under certain terms and conditions, and other terms and conditions.

Commonly used debt-type quasi-equity financing instruments include subordinated loans, income-sharing notes, convertible loans, convertible income-sharing notes, subordinated convertible income-sharing notes, convertible loans with call option, zero coupon convertible income-sharing notes, and others. Depending on what is allowed under local laws and regulations, such variations may include a preagreed rate of return on the original investment, which would be calculated in accordance with specific formulas that are included in the investment agreements.

A WORD OF CAUTION

The above discussions of alternative structures of equity and debt financing are provided to assist your planning process and help you gain a basic understanding of these topics. They are not exhaustive in their coverage of the many different ways in which equity and/or debt financing can be designed.

As a receiver of investments and the potential obligor of a put agreement or similar agreements, you will need to take extreme care to learn the full scope of the potential consequences, both financial and nonfinancial, of any arrangements before agreeing to them. Consulting legal experts on these matters early on can save you from spending time and effort in negotiating arrangements that may prove to be unworkable under the applicable laws.

6

Marketing Your Facility

If You Build It, Make Sure They Come

With all of the complexities involved in building a health care facility, project teams are constantly forced to deal with short-term project issues that must be resolved by the next deadline. As a result, priority usually goes to construction issues and other decisions that have a visible impact on physical progress and spending. Focusing on costs, both during construction and once operations begin, is clearly critical. Yet it is equally imperative to pay attention to how your hospital will generate revenues.

A newly completed hospital gets some publicity when it starts up operation, but continuing to build a good reputation and attract patients requires a well-structured marketing plan. All too often, physicians and first-time entrepreneurs are not aware of this important aspect and believe that building a state-of-the-art health care facility is enough to attract customers. Your hospital may indeed offer a variety of attractive and unique patient services, but simply making these services available will not guarantee that your facility can operate at sufficient capacity to produce reasonable profits for your investors in the long term or even break even financially in the short term.

The term "marketing" is often used interchangeably with "advertising" or "sales promotion." However, marketing refers to a broad range of activities that are undertaken to influence the target audience to have a positive view of the products, services, and brand names being marketed and, ultimately, to choose to buy them.

Developing and Refining Your Marketing Strategy

Successfully marketing your hospital depends on clearly defining the what, who, when, where, and how of your business strategy. These five key elements, discussed in more detail below, are interrelated. For example, the choice of a target audience will help to determine which particular services to focus on at any given point in your marketing campaign.

Although you need to develop a careful marketing plan, the plan should not be rigid. The first component will be the definition of the project's concept and mission statement, as discussed in chapter 2. Beyond that, however, elements such as the content, target audience, and time frame for the marketing activities all need to be reviewed and adjusted regularly as the hospital's planning and construction advance. After the hospital opens for business, the marketing plan will still need continuous adjustment in light of operational changes, technological advances, and patient and staff feedback, as well as any new information concerning market demand or competition.

What Should You Market?

Your marketing strategy will have two constant goals: to make your hospital known to the public and to attract as many paying patients as possible. Before getting into details of how your marketing program can be structured, you must carry out research on the country's laws and regulations concerning marketing and advertisements.

You might consider structuring the content of your marketing strategy in two main components. The first is to communicate what your hospital stands for and what it seeks to achieve, thus establishing a permanent image and "brand" for the hospital. Branding has to be consistent with, and reflective of, the vision, core values, and mission (some people refer to these as the "brand DNA") that you and your partners will determine for the hospital. The second component is to focus on one or more services offered by your hospital, a strategic decision that will shift over time while maintaining consistency with the first component.

The efforts to establish a brand for your hospital will aim to create confidence among prospective patients that they will receive the best care possible when they come to your hospital and that your hospital is best suited to meet their needs. The fact that well-known or well-qualified doctors practice at your hospital will therefore be one of the critical components of a successful branding effort. Accreditation by recognized international bodies may also be helpful. Messages related to branding have to be communicated consistently and continuously over a relatively long period in a manner that is both culturally appropriate and memorable. The content of the marketing program related to image and branding will probably not change much over time, unless there is a drastic change in the scope of the hospital's operations. The delivery mechanism, however, may undergo changes.

For the second component of your marketing strategy, you will focus on a "strategic" department, service, or treatment that is important to building up your hospital's reputation and revenues. To a large extent, these high-profile services will have been determined during the prefeasibility analysis (chapter 3) and the feasibility analysis (chapter 4). For example, you might focus on the cardiovascular department, emphasizing that it is led by the best-known heart doctor in the country or in the community. Or you could highlight the oncology department's state-of-the-art cancer treatments.

The strategic focus will likely shift over time. You may choose to highlight one or two services for a certain period of time and then switch the focus to other services later. For example, you might choose to publicize a unique and possibly high-priced service that you expect to be low-volume, and later shift the spotlight to services that you expect to be high-volume and high revenue generators.

To Whom Should You Market?

The next question to consider is who will be the target audience(s). The answer may differ for each of the two components of the marketing strategy discussed above. With respect to the first component, the hospital's image, the message needs to go out to a broad range of people including potential patients, health care professionals, government regulators, insurance companies, patient and environmental advocacy groups, pharmaceutical companies, and equipment suppliers. For the second component, specific services, the most obvious target audience would be potential patients, but probably specific groups of patients, depending upon the service you choose to market. Both components should be developed with a full understanding of the unique structure and characteristics of the health care market (box 6.1).

The choice of a target audience will also depend on the patient referral system and insurance programs that exist in the country. Even though patients will be your hospital's primary and most visible clients, they are seldom the only, or the ultimate, decision makers when it comes to choosing which hospital, physician, or clinic to visit and which services to purchase. For each service offered, the mix of decision makers will vary. For example, highly complex procedures such as a liver transplant are very expensive and can only be done in highly specialized facilities. The decision on where to get a liver transplant will depend on the referring physician's relationships and on his or her perceptions

> **Box 6.1   Unique Characteristics of the Health Care Market**
>
> The health care market differs from other markets in several important ways. First, there is frequently a three-way divide between the consumers of services (patients), the providers of services (medical personnel), and the decision makers who pay for the services (employees of national insurance funds or private insurance companies). Second, the consumer/patient typically has little ability to evaluate the quality of the services offered, either before or after the services are provided. Third, the consumer/patient is often unable to shop around and compare prices for medical services. Pricing information may be difficult to obtain in advance, and the patient who is ill or injured seldom has the time or ability to do much research. The patient may not even know what medical services are needed until he or she is already in a physician's consultation room.
>
> To illustrate: When you want to buy a new home audio system, you can visit several stores, listen to the equipment to compare sound quality, and gather price information. Based on this research, you can choose whether to buy, what to buy, and where to buy. But when you are ill, you might visit a physician and he or she will make a decision as to what medical services or products you need and when and where you will receive them. You have little ability to compare the technical quality of the indicated service—say, heart surgery—across different physicians and hospitals, or to shop around in advance for the best price. Often the physician who orders the service or medication may not know the price, and he or she almost certainly does not know how much of the price is covered by your insurance plan and how much you will pay out of pocket.
>
> In the new knowledge economy, some patients are becoming more informed on medical matters with the help of information channels such as the Internet. These informed patients are able to take a more active part in making decisions about their health care purchases. One result of this trend in the United States has been the increase in direct-to-consumer advertisements in the pharmaceutical industry.
>
> Nonetheless, because of the way the health care market is structured, use of a particular hospital will depend heavily on choices made by physicians and other health care providers. Here the referral system stands as a barrier to entry. Physicians may be bound to other competing hospitals by contractual obligations, bilateral referral systems, personal relationships, or force of habit, and this will determine where they send their patients for services. You, as the entrepreneur, need to carefully research how the referral system works and how your hospital can become a part of it, early in the process of planning your hospital. Failure to pay sufficient attention to this matter can have significant negative effects on your hospital's performance during the crucial first few years.
>
> All of these intrinsic characteristics of the health care market need to be taken into account when defining your marketing strategy. You must find out what drives the decision making with regard to consumption of each service your health care facility will offer and design your marketing strategy accordingly. Although many factors in health care decision making are beyond patients' control, the perceptions of patients and their family and friends about competing institutions can still affect the final decision on which hospital to visit. Health care providers, too, may be influenced by your hospital's reputation when they make referrals. Thus there is ample scope for marketing efforts to influence the flow of patients to your facility.

of the quality of the hospital's facility and staff; on the patient's perceptions of the hospital's advantages, such as location; and on the payer's reimbursement mechanism. Understanding how these decisions are made and how they can be influenced in your hospital's favor depends on understanding the structure and inner workings of your country's health care system.

An effective marketing program, therefore, also needs to build trust among medical professionals in your hospital's ability to provide the services they want for their patients. Compared to marketing activities directed to patients, marketing aimed at physicians will be quite technical, and you will need well-trained staff so that they can provide physicians with sufficient information. In addition, you could design a visiting doctors' program at the hospital as well as conferences, seminars, and other events targeted to medical professionals.

In addition to referring doctors, various other people are also likely to influence the patient's decision on which hospital to use, or they may even make the decision for the patient. Family members, friends, colleagues, industry experts, and so on may all be influential. Therefore, when you promote a specific service offered by your hospital, you will want to prepare and deliver a message that effectively reaches specific groups of people who are likely to weigh in on patients' decisions regarding which hospital to visit.

When Should You Market?

Development of a marketing strategy should begin early in the overall process of planning for your hospital. As your project gets underway, and especially as you complete your feasibility analysis and begin discussions with potential financiers, you may come across opportunities to talk with local journalists or people in the health care industry. At certain points you may wish to host a reception, such as when you are ready to publicize the schematic drawings of the hospital's design or when you announce a significant commitment from a financial partner. You should regard every such event as a part of your marketing program and plan to use the forum to get your message across.

In terms of what is communicated, the message sent out when the first brick is laid during construction will be different from the message projected when thousands of patients have already been treated in your facility. It is useful to examine the timing of your marketing strategy in relation to the project's phases. During the feasibility analysis and the facility planning and design stages, your marketing efforts will focus on broadening awareness of your project concept and mission among potential investors and financiers, relevant regulators, the physician community, and the insurance and pharmaceutical industries. You want to gain approval and buy-in of your project's concept among these stakeholders.

As your project plans are put into action, coinciding with the construction phase, the awareness campaign will be expanded to reach the broad public, building up their eagerness to visit the hospital when it opens its doors. In the preopening preparation period, marketing will become more specific, focusing on priority services and patient groups. Such activities will intensify during the first 12 months of the hospital's operation. After your facility has been operating for over a year, your marketing efforts will become much more dynamic as you seek to manage the reputation you are developing in the marketplace based on real customer experiences and feedback, and reinforce the messages you want to communicate.

Where Should You Market?

The geographic focus of your marketing strategy may be local, regional, national, international, or some combination of these. How you decide to answer the previous "what" and "who" questions will directly affect where you should conduct your marketing activities. The competitive advantages of your business model at each geographic level and the cost-effectiveness of marketing at each level must be considered as well.

How Should You Market?

The question of how to implement your marketing program has three aspects: delivery mechanisms, tools for development of a comprehensive marketing program, and organization of the marketing activities (or organization for implementation of the marketing program).

Delivery mechanisms

Once you have crafted a message, you must decide how to deliver it. Your answers to the four questions discussed above (what, to whom, when, and where to market) will influence, and be influenced by, the choice of delivery mechanisms. There is a wide variety available, including promotional events and programs, advertisements, and public relations outreach. You should understand how these mechanisms differ in their scope and cost so that you can determine the optimal combination of activities at a given time and within your budget. As noted above, you should first find out what if any constraints are imposed by local laws and regulations, as some countries do not allow advertisements by health care facilities.

Promotional events and programs have the dual goal of stimulating demand for the target product or service and enhancing the image and brand name of the producer or provider of the service. They could include, for example, giveaways

---

Box 6.2   A Marketing Innovation: Franco-Vietnamese Hospital's Medical Card

By the time the Franco-Vietnamese Hospital in Ho Chi Minh City, Vietnam opened its doors to the public, it had launched a number of advertisements through radio, magazines, and other media to increase the public's awareness of its existence. It had also implemented several other types of marketing and public relations programs, including numerous receptions and press conferences. However, the hospital was still looking for another way to spread the word quickly.

Hospital developers had learned during the feasibility analysis that most Vietnamese do not obtain regular health checkups. They decided to encourage people to come to the hospital by offering checkups at an affordable price under a special promotional program. A person or a family purchases a membership card for a fixed amount that is valid for one year and entitles the cardholder to a number of free consultations and screenings, as well as emergency care. The smart-looking card bears the name, logo, location, and contact information of the hospital, as well as the name and photo of the cardholder.

The card program quickly became popular. The hospital has since expanded the program to include four different categories of packaged services at different prices, including discounts on hospitalization costs, so that the program now serves almost as a quasi-medical insurance program.

In addition to benefiting individual cardholders, the program has contributed to the public good by making early preventive medical care available to the public at affordable prices. The cardholders who come to the hospital for checkups tell their friends and families about the hospital's facilities and atmosphere. The medical exams provide an opportunity to identify patients who need additional medical services. And sales of the cards bring in cash receipts for the hospital before costs are actually incurred.

For more information: Franco-Vietnamese Hospital, http://www.fvhospital.com/.

---

or discounts on selected products or services, such as a one-day free immunization campaign. Other examples include celebratory events such as receptions, informational events such as conferences and workshops, displays of posters urging people to be screened for a certain disease, showings of videos or movies, and distribution of informational brochures and flyers. In addition, published materials such as quarterly newsletters distributed to doctors in the referral network can serve as an effective marketing tool. Many promotional activities can be carried out in partnership with other institutions that share common objectives with your hospital or that expect to gain benefits by doing joint activities. An example of an innovative promotion is the medical card program introduced by the Franco-Vietnamese Hospital, which combines promotion of the hospital's services with aspects of an insurance program (box 6.2).

Advertisements aim to increase the awareness of, and the desire to purchase, target products or services. They often address a mass audience by means of the mass media. Because advertising messages are widely disseminated, it is especially important to ensure that their content is accurate, and the potential for legal issues needs to be carefully examined before an advertisement is approved. Cultural and religious sensitivities should be considered when designing advertisements.

Public relations efforts seek to deliver the same messages by informing a third party, such as a journalist, about a product, service, or facility being promoted. The aim is to have your message featured in a newspaper or magazine article or a television or radio news report or interview that is presented as general information and does not appear to be intentionally promoting a particular product. The provider of the product or service usually does not appear as the provider of the information. Unlike advertising, public relations outreach usually does not involve payment to the media; however, you also have less control over the message that appears, or even whether anything appears at all. For instance, you might send a press release to a newspaper on the opening of your new hospital in hopes that a reporter will write an article about the opening as an event of interest to the community. Or members of your medical staff might offer technical expertise to a television journalist doing a report on new trends in the treatment of cardiovascular disease; if you are lucky, your hospital will be mentioned and your staff doctors quoted by name. Being associated with such news coverage is an effective way to increase the community's awareness of your facility.

Marketing tools

In order to formulate an effective overall marketing program, you will need to have at your disposal a few essential tools, including a database, market studies, and satisfaction surveys. Through consultation with your core project team and marketing professionals who have experience in the health care industry, you and your partners can determine what kinds of data will be useful in developing your marketing program. The specific data set that you will collect will center on your target population and the marketing activities you are directing toward them. The database has to be designed to accommodate sufficient data inputs relating to current and potential patient groups, market segments, target corporate entities, content and frequency of specific marketing activities, and so on. Once developed, the database has to be updated regularly.

You should carry out the first market study or survey before your hospital is constructed, during the feasibility analysis stage. Once the hospital opens and begins full operations, market studies should be conducted at regular intervals in order to better understand the needs of your hospital's target population, the effectiveness of your marketing program, and your hospital's image and reputation in the community.

The most reliable first-hand data will come from client satisfaction surveys. Such surveys should be conducted among hospitalized inpatients, outpatients who visit for consultations only, referring doctors, and the hospital's own staff. The questions asked should be ones that help identify specific actions needed for improvement of the hospital's services. Patients may be reluctant to fill out questionnaires for several reasons, including fear of potential repercussions if they give negative answers or simply lack of experience in responding to surveys. Therefore, you need to think about how to maximize the number of surveys completed as well as how to ensure that their content is useful. Your hospital's marketing department and its quality assurance department should coordinate closely on all aspects of the work concerning satisfaction surveys.

ORGANIZATIONAL ASPECTS

In deciding how to carry out your marketing activities, you might consider contracting with an external marketing agency rather than having your own marketing department. This option has drawbacks, however, such as lack of flexibility and control over content and delivery, possible delays or inefficiencies, and high costs. Some hospitals prefer to differentiate activities related to branding and image building, development of relationships with referral doctors and industry professionals, knowledge sharing, community service, and so on, from sales promotion and advertisements. In such case, a separate department for business development may be established to manage the former group of activities.

While there are many marketing possibilities, it is easy to make mistakes in formulating and implementing a marketing strategy. For example, the target audience groups may not be selected properly, the artwork may use inappropriate images or colors, posters may be posted in the wrong places, radio messages may be broadcast at the wrong time, and so forth. Such blunders mean lost opportunities for the activity to generate the intended results and loss of limited budget resources. Although it is not easy to do, a return-on-expense analysis or a cost-effectiveness analysis may prove helpful in determining which marketing activities are best from a resource allocation perspective.

Building and Maintaining the Hospital's Reputation

Building up and maintaining a good image and reputation for your hospital will be critical to ensuring its long-term success. The first step toward that goal is recognizing the many different stakeholders whose perceptions and opinions can influence your hospital's reputation. The other dimension is the quality of services provided by the facility and the level of fees charged.

Different Stakeholders and Their Perceptions

In addition to patients and their families, many different groups have a stake in seeing that your hospital is operated well and meets their expectations. They include your staff, members of your corporate governance structure, your professional partners and collaborators, government authorities, consumer and environmental advocacy groups, and members of the community where your hospital will be located. You will need to understand what is most important to each of these groups in terms of shaping their perception of your hospital and what specific actions or events (which may or may not be under the hospital's control) could have a positive or negative impact on these perceptions (box 6.3).

For patients and their families, knowing that they can receive high-quality service safely at affordable prices will be the most important aspect. In this regard, patients want to know that your hospital has the best physicians and well-trained, caring, and friendly staff. Patients tend to be particularly demanding of value for their money when they are paying for the services with their own funds. Your medical personnel and other staff may attach the most importance to the availability of dependable medical equipment, clearly stated operating rules that are enforced consistently, a pleasant working environment, and ample training and other benefits. To your professional partners and collaborators, your hospital's steady growth, business opportunities, and innovative working

---

Box 6.3 Targeted Marketing Efforts: The Apollo Hospitals Group

The Apollo Hospitals Group is the largest private health care provider in Asia. Its marketing efforts incorporate seminars, workshops, online content, media outreach, and public relations work. The business has special strategies for reaching out to doctors, patients, and corporations.

Doctors: The Apollo Group conducts educational seminars and workshops for doctors and has created an interactive Web site on hospital infrastructure and the latest medical techniques for physicians. Apollo relies on media and public relations to instill confidence in its health care services by recognizing its doctors.

Patients: Apollo hospitals reach out to consumers by offering medical education and awareness sessions and organizing special events on designated "health days." Additionally, Apollo collaborates with travel services and resort operators to offer medical tourism packages to overseas patients.

Corporations: Apollo markets special plans for corporations and offers corporate employees cardiac screening and health checkups as well as stress-relieving programs such as meditation.

Sources: "Making Health Accessible," *Hindu Business Line*, June 13, 2002; "Hospital Marketing Comes of Age," *Express Healthcare Management*, January 15–31, 2005.

relationships will lead to favorable perceptions. Your suppliers, such as pharmaceutical companies, will look for reasonable lead times on orders and for timely payment of bills. Regulators will have a good impression if your hospital always passes its various inspections, has no medical accidents, and observes all relevant laws and regulations.

Often perceptions are built on chance encounters, occasional observations, or word of mouth. These are just as important as repeated first-hand direct encounters. In the case of a health care facility, one medical accident can damage overnight the image that the facility has carefully developed over years.

A Patient-Centered Culture

Of all the stakeholder groups mentioned above, patients are the ones whom it is most crucial to please. Quality of care and medical outcomes are the most important influences on patient perceptions and on the reputation of a health care facility in general.

Three aspects of a patient-centered culture are a patient service charter, patient-centered procedures, and patient-sensitive medical and administrative staff. Formulating a patient service charter, which usually extends your mission statement and your marketing messages, is a useful way to explicitly inform your patients, partners, and staff about the operating standards your facility has set for itself. These standards can cover all aspects of your services, even such minor matters as how many times the telephone will be permitted to ring before it is answered or how many days patients must wait between requesting an appointment and seeing a physician in a nonemergency situation. All written documentation concerning clinical procedures, medical outcomes, standards for quality care, and the quality control system should be prepared with a patient-centered perspective so that a patient-centered approach can be put in practice when such standards and procedures are followed in daily operation. Furthermore, sensitivity to patients has to be built into your hospital's corporate culture and operating policies. This will require regular training programs for medical and nonmedical staff.

Finally, as noted above, obtaining feedback from patients and their families should be an integral part of your patient management system. Patients in general tend not to complain to their health care providers when they feel dissatisfied. Instead, they vocalize their unhappiness to family members, friends, and colleagues. Your challenge is to put in place a system that gives patients and their families an opportunity to voice their dissatisfaction through established channels; this will help you uncover and resolve potential issues before they disrupt the hospital's operations and blemish its reputation. A well-designed feedback system will help the hospital understand patients' perceptions and which aspects of the hospital experience affect their perceptions most. It can also reveal which of the hospital's services are seen to be of acceptable quality and which need improvement. You can then develop appropriate corrective actions for the problems identified. Providing patients and their families with follow-up responses to the issues they have raised is very important to a meaningful patient management system.

7

Facility Planning and Design

Time to Start Drawings

Before you can see your dream take detailed shape on paper, a number of crucial elements must be in place. You and your partners should have gained confidence in the project's potential viability based on the feasibility analysis, which will still be underway. You should have raised at least 5–10 percent of the estimated total project cost. And you should have hired—or at a minimum, should have identified—a core team of professionals, persons who will play the critical roles discussed below.

In addition, you should have identified a land parcel of a condition and size suitable for your hospital project and obtained a substantial and legally binding commitment from the owner of the land.

Translating ideas into a specific design and then into a real-life operating structure is an exciting leap. But before you can break ground for construction, every aspect of the hospital needs to be carefully planned. In addition to ensuring that the hospital's physical setting is consistent with your project concept, conducting detailed work on the facility design will be key to obtaining realistic estimates of the project cost. The early stage of work on the hospital's design, up to the conceptual or preliminary drawing stage, is a part of the feasibility analysis. As discussed in chapter 4, a feasibility analysis cannot be fully completed or finalized without considering essential elements of a hospital's design. These in turn may have a broad range of implications, including a large impact on the project's cost estimates.

Depending on the specific circumstances of the country and locality where your hospital will be located, you may wish to explore the possibility of remodeling an existing hospital. If this is an option, keep in mind that many hospitals in developing countries are housed in very old buildings, which may be in poor repair and which differ greatly from modern buildings in functional design. In addition, existing buildings may not accommodate the installation of up-to-date communication and IT systems and sophisticated medical equipment. Therefore, any decision to undertake remodeling or adaptation of an existing, presumably old, hospital must be examined carefully in order to obtain a realistic cost estimate.

Three major pitfalls can affect the facility design stage. One is failure to invest sufficiently in development of a thorough feasibility analysis, as described in chapter 4. The other two are failure to retain an architectural firm experienced in designing health care facilities and failure to build a team of knowledgeable individuals or organizations and involve them closely in the design process. The latter two areas are discussed in more detail in the sections below.

The Facility Design and Planning Team

As you launch the design stage, you will need to assemble a larger team of professionals whose knowledge and experience can help ensure that the design and construction plans are realistic and affordable.[10] In addition to you and your partners (that is, the project owners) and the project director as discussed in chapter 2, your planning team ideally will include the following members:

- Chief executive officer or medical planner or medical director (also called director of clinical operations)
- Project manager (an individual or professional firm with sufficient experience in working with international clients, preferably in developing countries)
- Architect(s), design engineers, and interior designers
- Consultant for the site and geotechnical analysis
- Specialty consultants who will cover such areas as biomedical engineering, acoustics, food services, IT systems, and materials management
- Construction manager (see chapter 9 for a discussion of the construction manager's role)
- Medical equipment planner, who should have come on board during the project's feasibility analysis stage
- Director of nursing
- Chief financial officer

---

10. This section draws on information and feedback provided by Dr. Joel Nobel of ECRI; Dr. Jean-Marcel Guillon, chairman of Franco-Vietnamese Hospital; Douglas Heilser, founder of META Associates (now part of Parsons META); and Daniel Olphie III of Parsons META.

A brief description of the role of some of these key members is provided below.

Chief Executive Officer

You will need to identify and hire a chief executive officer (CEO) for the hospital by the time you start the design and construction plans. Once the building is physically completed and opens its doors, the CEO will become responsible for day-to-day operation of the hospital. But the CEO should also participate in the hospital's design stage, because the physical set-up of the facility and the composition of the professional team will be key to his or her ability to successfully manage the hospital. By weighing in at this stage, the CEO will help ensure that the layout of the facility, the construction details, and key equipment and fixtures are of the type and quality necessary to enable the hospital staff to function effectively and efficiently. At the same time, the CEO will have the opportunity to understand the flexibilities and constraints, if any, of the hospital's physical setting, so that he or she can take these aspects into account in planning the hospital's daily operations later on. For this reason, the CEO has to be a person who has sufficient knowledge and experience not only of the daily operation of hospitals but also of the design and planning, construction management, and preopening preparations.

The reality in many developing countries, however, is that it is very difficult to find professionals who meet such requirements. Even in developed countries, it is not easy to find a CEO who has this range of experience. In such circumstances you may need to find a way to retain on a part-time basis, in the early stage, a person who you believe can eventually become your hospital's CEO with responsibility mainly for business and management issues, and support him or her by finding someone else who can play the role of a medical planner (see below).

One of the most critical functions that the CEO often has to perform is to resist the unrealistic or impractical wishes of the project's sponsors/owners—that is, you and your partners—and of the physicians. As noted earlier, project sponsors are often tempted to build a bigger and better facility than they can afford financially and/or can manage. Physicians, for their part, tend to favor their own specialties, with limited regard for the impact on the hospital's overall finances, planning, construction, and, later, daily operations. Therefore, the CEO needs to be someone who has a grasp of the full scope of what it will take to make the hospital become a reality.

As noted earlier, the CEO should come on board as early as possible so that he or she can become fully familiar with the project's concept and vision and planning details. This will also allow the CEO to establish operating policies and procedures and provide consistency in day-to-day management and leadership, both for the hospital's staff as they come on board and for the project's external team members (such as the construction contractors, medical equipment planner, suppliers, and so forth). In any case, a full-time CEO should be hired at least one year before the hospital's opening. If possible, the remuneration package of the CEO should be structured in a way that combines a fixed-amount annual or monthly salary with an annual bonus.

Project Manager

A project manager plays a central role during the planning, construction, and opening stages to ensure that all necessary steps are undertaken in a timely and effective manner. This person or firm assists the project's owners and project director in the evaluation and selection of architects, contractors, and consultants; schedules work programs; coordinates work among all member of the extended project team; and monitors progress in all aspects of the process. The project manager should have sufficient knowledge about all critical technical matters and should also understand the business, social, and cultural aspects of the work environment. Obviously, good managerial capabilities are essential, as are demonstrated integrity and accountability to the project sponsors. If a project is relatively small, an individual with sufficient technical knowledge and managerial capabilities (for example, the project director or the CEO) may be able to carry out this function successfully. In the case of a secondary or tertiary hospital, the project manager most likely needs to be a professional firm that has sufficient experience and a large pool of professionals that can be mobilized to ensure high-quality service.

Medical Planner

If you have not been able to find a CEO who has the qualifications noted above by the time you are ready to start work on the hospital's design, you may need to recruit a medical planner for this stage of the project. An experienced medical planner typically has a broad understanding of what it takes to design, construct, and open a new hospital in terms of clinical, organizational, logistical, and management needs, and can provide guidance to the hospital's planning and design team on practical, logistical, and functional matters. The main distinction between a CEO and a medical planner is that the medical planner provides expertise during a hospital's planning and design stage without any expectation or commitment that he or she will later become responsible for the hospital's management.

If you have difficulty identifying a qualified medical planner, you will at least need to have a medical director or director of clinical operations (DCO). A DCO is a professional who specializes in managing all aspects of the day-to-day clinical affairs of a hospital, including some level of administrative tasks. In the absence of a qualified CEO or medical planner, a DCO can provide critically needed input regarding the hospital's planned clinical operations during the facility design stage. If you have a CEO or a medical planner on board during the hospital's planning stage, a DCO should be hired at least six months before the hospital opens.

Architect

The facility design work will be led by your architect or architects. Ideally, you will hire an architectural firm, which can bring a team of professionals headed by a lead architect to complete your project. You need to identify a firm that has experience in successfully designing and developing at least several medium-size secondary or tertiary care hospitals, if that is the type of facility you are building. It is important that the firm have specific experience with health care facilities and not just experience with other large facilities such as hotels, which resemble hospitals in some respects but are entirely different in many critical areas.

In many developing countries it is difficult to find local architectural firms that have solid hospital experience. In such situations, you may need to look for either a foreign architectural firm or a foreign individual architect with experience in designing hospitals, preferably in a neighboring country. You can twin this foreign firm or architect with a local firm or architect whose experience does not include hospitals. Teaming up foreign and local architects will help ensure that aspects unique to the country and region where your hospital will be located are properly addressed. However, this foreign/local team approach also entails risks: many unexpected events can occur and the planned outcomes may not be achieved due to misunderstandings, language barriers, distance, personality clashes, and the possible lack of commitment of the foreign architect.

Switching to a new architect after preliminary design work has already been completed can be disruptive and costly. Therefore, it is better to spend some extra time and money at the early stage to identify an architectural firm or a team of architects that has the right experience, that can build trust and a comfortable working relationship with you and your partners, and that will make a commitment to complete your project. In some countries you may not have many choices. In those circumstances it is even more important for you to identify the right architectural team or firm by contacting various architectural firms both at home and abroad. You can also ask for references from existing hospitals and from other sources such as medical equipment suppliers and independent advisory firms.

Medical Equipment Planner

A medical equipment planner is an expert whose role is uncommon in many developing countries. However, such a person or firm provides important expertise and objective advice to project developers who are faced with the task of selecting complex and sophisticated medical equipment. Because the function is highly specialized, it may not be easy to find an experienced medical equipment planner in the country where your hospital will be located. However, given the large amounts of money at stake in purchasing big-ticket medical equipment, allocating a part of your limited development budget to finding an experienced equipment planner could be a wise investment.

An experienced consulting firm may often be the best choice for the medical equipment planning role. Dealing with medical equipment requires knowledge and expertise in a range of highly specialized areas, including surgical operations and clinical laboratories. An advisory firm typically has a large team of professionals with experience in different areas concerning the planning, procurement, installation, and postinstallation management of medical equipment; these individuals can be assigned to the project as a team. In addition, a well-established advisory firm normally has databases that can provide much of the information needed for the schematic design stage. Try to identify an independent firm that is not associated with equipment manufacturers or suppliers and that does not receive any finder's fee or supplier's commission.

Experienced medical equipment planners have detailed knowledge about the technical and business features of various medical equipment models and about trends in the development of new technologies. They also know the leading medical equipment manufacturers and suppliers. After helping to identify a suitable set of medical equipment items for your hospital, the medical equipment planner can also manage the process of preparing specifications and can review, if applicable, the tender submissions from equipment suppliers or manufacturers in response to request for bids under a competitive bidding process. The planning team can then help you make the final selection based on previously established selection criteria (see chapter 8) and ensure that the equipment's installation is done properly.

As noted in chapter 4, a qualified medical equipment planner should be on board at the feasibility analysis stage and should be a core member of the project team throughout the development and construction of the hospital.

Director of Nursing

If possible, the hospital's physical setting should be planned with full participation of the person who will eventually become your hospital's director of nursing (DON). The DON's input is very important in the hospital design stage because an experienced nurse knows how the space and layout of a hospital affects the operations of the nursing staff. Nurses undertake tasks that are different from those of physicians and these tasks have specific space and functional needs, especially with respect to the relationship between patient rooms and nursing stations, as well as infection control.

Chief Financial Officer

A chief financial officer (CFO) has expertise that goes beyond that of an auditor or accountant. In addition to being responsible for budgeting, financial analysis, and financial reporting, the CFO takes the lead in deciding how the hospital's construction and operations will be financed. He or she chooses the optimum mix of different financing instruments and negotiates terms and conditions of financing with each financial partner. A qualified CFO should be knowledgeable about how banks work and about the various financing instruments and their usual terms and conditions, as well as flexibilities that may be possible in negotiating them. He or she is also expected to be familiar with how bond and stock markets work and with the role of investment banks. The ideal CFO either has an extensive network of contacts in the banking and financial consulting industries or is capable of developing such contacts.

Like the CEO, an experienced CFO should have the ability to resist the wishes of project sponsors/owners by articulating the financial consequences of different choices regarding the hospital's design and construction and other major cost items. This will help you and your partners make decisions that are within the limits of the amount of financing you can obtain. The CFO should also be familiar with how to build a good financial projection model and should be able to guide and monitor a financial consultant or a junior staff person in building the projection model, if necessary.

Hiring a full-time CFO at this early stage may not be necessary or cost-efficient. If you have not been able to identify a qualified CFO, or if you wish to hire a qualified CFO later (but not less than 10–12 months before the hospital's opening), you will need someone who can fill this function during the early stages of your hospital project. In this case you could consider retaining an external accounting firm to handle all matters concerning budgeting, accounting, financial reporting, and recordkeeping, while getting help from an experienced financial consultant in obtaining financing.

Space and Functional Programming

The essential first steps in designing your hospital are to estimate how much space can be created and in what form on the piece of land you have secured and how the space will be allocated for each function to be carried out in your hospital. As you and your partners make tentative decisions on what types of treatments and procedures your hospital will offer, based on the outcome of market analysis and research, you should analyze the implications of these decisions for the hospital's overall design and space requirements. The physical setting of the facility, interior as well as exterior, should help convey the hospital's vision and mission in an architecturally appealing and functionally efficient way.

Considerations for functional allocation of space include such basic and critical questions as how many operating rooms, patient rooms, and laboratories will be installed and where they will be located. Also to be considered are the number and location of examining and procedure rooms, inventory rooms, administrative offices, nursing stations, staff relaxation rooms, patient waiting areas, conference rooms, and lavatories, as well as the pharmacy, kitchens, laundry room, cafeteria, and gift shop. The design needs to take into account the installation of major medical equipment, communication and IT systems, mechanical and electrical systems, and utilities such as gas supply systems. Each procedure and treatment, as well as each nonmedical service for the comfort and convenience of patients and visitors, has to be analyzed for its logistical and space needs, taking into account the relationships among the various departments and the pattern of physical movements of people, equipment, and supplies. In addition, steps necessary to ensure the safety and environmental soundness of the hospital's operation, as well as the needs for future expansion, have to be considered. To the extent possible, consider the possibility of outsourcing certain ancillary services before designing space for in-house provision of all services. A suggested approach to programming the functions and operations of each service or department is provided in appendix O.

When estimating the amount of space needed for delivering each treatment or procedure, cultural and social customs and preferences that influence people's behavior need to be considered carefully. For example, making separate spaces available for males and females may be more important in certain regions and countries than in others. You can benefit from the results of a well-planned market research or consumer survey to understand and identify social and cultural factors.

Conceptual (Preliminary) Design

As the team makes decisions about the services to be provided and the specific functions and departments that will deliver such services, the architect will start to create initial conceptual drawings of the hospital, working in consultation with you and your partners, the CEO or medical planner, the medical equipment planner, and other members of the planning team discussed above.

It is important in this phase to remain flexible, yet keep changes to the necessary minimum. Modifications to the conceptual drawings may be needed to reflect new information about the market, such as news of other hospitals under construction or planned; the outcome of discussions that you and your partners have with potential sources of financing; or simply a change in the way you and your partners conceive of the project. Revisions to drawings (or making new drawings) at the conceptual design stage will not cost as much as making such changes at the schematic design stage, discussed below. One of the most common causes of too many revisions is lack of necessary expertise in key areas at the time of drawing. While repeated changes to the conceptual design may be unavoidable because of events beyond your control, they can be minimized by making sure that the research and discussions preceding the drawings are sufficiently detailed and involve members of the planning team and physicians.

In addition, clear and logical thinking and consensus among you and your partners will be an important factor in this process. At this stage, each new conceptual design has to be subjected to a revision of cost estimates in order to develop a design that can be achieved at the lowest cost possible. However, in estimating costs the team should be mindful of the impact of each choice on the future operating costs of the hospital, not just the construction. What may appear to be cost-saving at the outset could lead to much higher continuing costs after the hospital begins operation.

Schematic Design

By the time a consensus is reached on a conceptual design that appears to be workable, the feasibility analysis should have been substantially completed. The first draft of a full-scope business plan can then be prepared to use in serious discussions with potential financial partners. You should obtain substantial evidence of commitment for amounts covering at least 50 percent of the total estimated project cost before starting the schematic drawings. "Substantial evidence" in this context would be a written expression of strong interest in financing the project. The schematic design stage will cost a considerable amount of money; therefore its timing should be determined carefully.

By this time you should have secured the land, and the geotechnical and other site-related tests should have been completed and reported so that you will know what if any issues exist and require remedial actions before construction. You will also have obtained various licenses and permits necessary to begin the design process in earnest. The hospital operating license is likely to be the last license obtained, as it is only available after the hospital's construction has been completed and the hospital has passed various inspections. As you move into the schematic design stage, the lead architect will usually act as the primary coordinator of design efforts, working closely with other members of the project team.

The drawings prepared during this stage will cover details of each floor and each functional area, both interior and exterior. They will show circulation patterns that reflect the flows of patients, physicians, nurses, visitors, and support personnel, along with various materials. Details of the interior design, engineering drawings, and specifications are generated during this stage. In addition, equipment and furnishings for the facility and patient care are planned on a room-by-room basis and aggregated and priced. An equipment list and a realistic budget for medical and other equipment will be prepared as the architectural schematics and room lists are being completed. For the exterior, the designs should consider parking space on the hospital's premises, the likelihood that new roads or other facilities will be built near the hospital, the access route from the main road to the hospital, the best option for locating the hospital's front side, space for gardens, and so on.

What is done during this stage will affect the efficiency of the hospital's physical setting and staff and its operating costs for years to come. For this reason, the schematic design needs to be developed with the greatest possible participation of structural, mechanical, and electrical engineers, as well as specialists in medical equipment, vertical transportation, materials management, waste management, food service, and laundry service. Later, in the design development phase, other specialists such as acoustic, communications, and IT engineers and interior designers will need to join the team. The architect usually identifies the various engineers and specialists needed for the project, although the final selection of the individuals or firms to be retained is made in consultation with you and your partners and the CEO and/or medical planner.

The schematic design package contains three-dimensional drawings, architectural models, and virtual facility tours. The schematic design drawings, combined with the plans for future expansion (see below), form the master plan for facility design. They also provide the basis for preparation of the even more detailed design development documents. The design development documents in turn form the basis for preparation of the construction documents, as discussed in chapter 9.

Consider Future Expansion

In many cases, a multistage building plan may be necessary. Provisions for future expansion should not be an afterthought but should be incorporated into the master plan and considered at each stage of site selection, site planning, department planning, and functional programming, as well as preparation of schematic design, so that future expansions can be undertaken without having to substantially modify various drawings. The phased development plan needs to show how the hospital can be expanded without disruption of current services, how each department can expand independently (and to what maximum size), and how new services or building elements can be added in a logical manner.

The approach to a staged development plan will depend largely upon the availability and price of land. Vertical expansions can be costly for a variety of reasons, including more up-front investments needed for foundations, structural strength, extra elevator shafts, and so forth. Such higher cost can be a significant burden on the hospital's finances, especially during the first five years of operation. Horizontal expansions are considered more desirable because they are easier to implement, less disruptive to ongoing operations, and less costly. However, horizontal expansions will entail higher land costs and higher energy costs in the long run because of the greater roof area. The benefits and constraints of each approach need to be evaluated carefully.

In preparing the phased development plans or expansion plans, you need to keep in mind the possibility that your hospital's needs will change. Many different factors may have an effect on future design and use of the hospital facilities: evolving patterns of disease, new treatments, changes in patient preferences and lifestyles, innovations in industrial and construction materials, and of course the tremendous ongoing advances in telecommunications, information systems, and technology. For example, in recent decades ambulatory services and outpatient centers have seen significant growth in many countries. This is a departure from the traditional focus on in-patient treatments and has reduced the number of patient rooms needed at many hospitals. A simpler example is the matter of parking space. In many developing countries the growth of car ownership has significantly exceeded expectations, resulting in a huge shortage of parking space in many urban areas; an expansion of your hospital would need to take this into account.

Cost Projections

As discussed in chapter 4, cost projections will undergo numerous revisions and updates as the work progresses on the feasibility analysis and the hospital design. At the early stage of the feasibility analysis, you will have made rough estimates of the total project cost based on cost per room or some other rule of thumb. As the work continues in the schematic design stage, the cost estimates will become more detailed and realistic than the initial estimates.

As the budget for construction-related costs is updated, it may have an impact on the financial projections, depending on the reasons for the updates. For example, if the construction budget is being revised because of changes to the hospital's facilities that will have a direct influence on its clinical operations—such as the number of operating rooms or installation of key medical equipment—these changes are likely to have considerable impact on the hospital's revenue and cash generation. On the other hand, if revisions are made that do not affect the hospital's essential elements, such as changes in the facility layout or in construction materials, these may have less impact on the overall financial projections.

8

Major Medical Equipment

Not Everyone Needs an MRI

In order to operate smoothly, a hospital needs a variety of equipment, tools, spare parts, and supplies, ranging from expensive medical equipment to a microwave oven for the kitchen. Full discussion of all issues concerning selection and procurement of medical and nonmedical equipment and supplies is beyond the scope of this chapter. We have therefore chosen to focus on major medical equipment with unit costs of over $25,000, particularly those items that could be considered "cornerstone" equipment, as these have the greatest potential impact on the construction and operation of a hospital. Depending on the hospital's concept and size, key medical equipment can account for 10–25 percent of the facility's total construction budget, excluding preopening costs and permanent working capital. Procurement of a complex, big-ticket item such as a computed tomography (CT) scan machine can have a significant impact on a hospital's image and on its financial performance.

There are many pitfalls concerning procurement, installation, and maintenance of major medical equipment. As discussed in chapters 7 and 9, it is essential to develop and integrate specifications for such equipment into the hospital design and construction planning. Well-timed and well-coordinated management of the selection, procurement, and installation processes will be critical to successful completion of the hospital's construction on schedule and within budget. The keys are to select the right equipment for your hospital, set a realistic timetable for procurement, pay attention to the terms and conditions of the purchase contract and related matters, make meticulous preparations for delivery and installation, and ensure adequate training for personnel who will use the equipment.

A Systematic Approach

In some developing countries, the choice of equipment and the terms and conditions of purchase are limited by which items can be imported and which global suppliers of medical equipment are active in the country. These and other constraints, such as the lack of an experienced medical equipment planner, often make it difficult or impractical for hospitals and entrepreneurs in developing countries to follow all of the steps and the logical sequence shown in figure 8.1.

Steps that should ideally occur in a sequence may instead occur simultaneously, and one step may influence the outcome of another. For example, depending on circumstances, you may need to conduct tentative negotiations regarding the terms and conditions of purchase while you and your partners are still trying to finalize the hospital's design. Depending on the results of these discussions with equipment suppliers and manufacturers (and/or their agents and brokers), it is conceivable that you and your partners may decide to modify the range of services that the hospital will provide.

You will need to do your own research and become aware of issues concerning medical equipment early in the planning process, well before you actually select any major medical equipment for purchase. During the planning process, it will be necessary to include in the discussions the principal physicians who are likely to practice at your hospital and who understand the functional needs of your hospital and the equipment being considered.

In countries where the distribution system is well developed, there are many agents and brokers specializing in medical equipment. An agent has an exclusive relationship with one or more medical equipment manufacturers. An agent, therefore, is likely to be more knowledgeable about his or her clients' products than about the products of other makers and will try to sell the equipment made by those clients. A broker is an independent distributor who handles products made by many different manufacturers. As such, a broker may be more knowledgeable than an agent about a broad range of products and may be a better source of information for a comparative analysis of different makes and models of equipment. To some extent, brokers may also be viewed as more neutral than agents when it comes to recommending one product or model over others. However, keep in mind that a broker may also have an incentive to push for sale of a particular model, depending on the amount of commissions or other incentives provided by different suppliers.

Selection Criteria

The selection of key medical equipment depends on many factors, including clinical and technological adequacy, supplier reliability, facility constraints, user

Figure 8.1   Step-by-Step Approach to Planning, Procurement, and Management of Medical Equipment

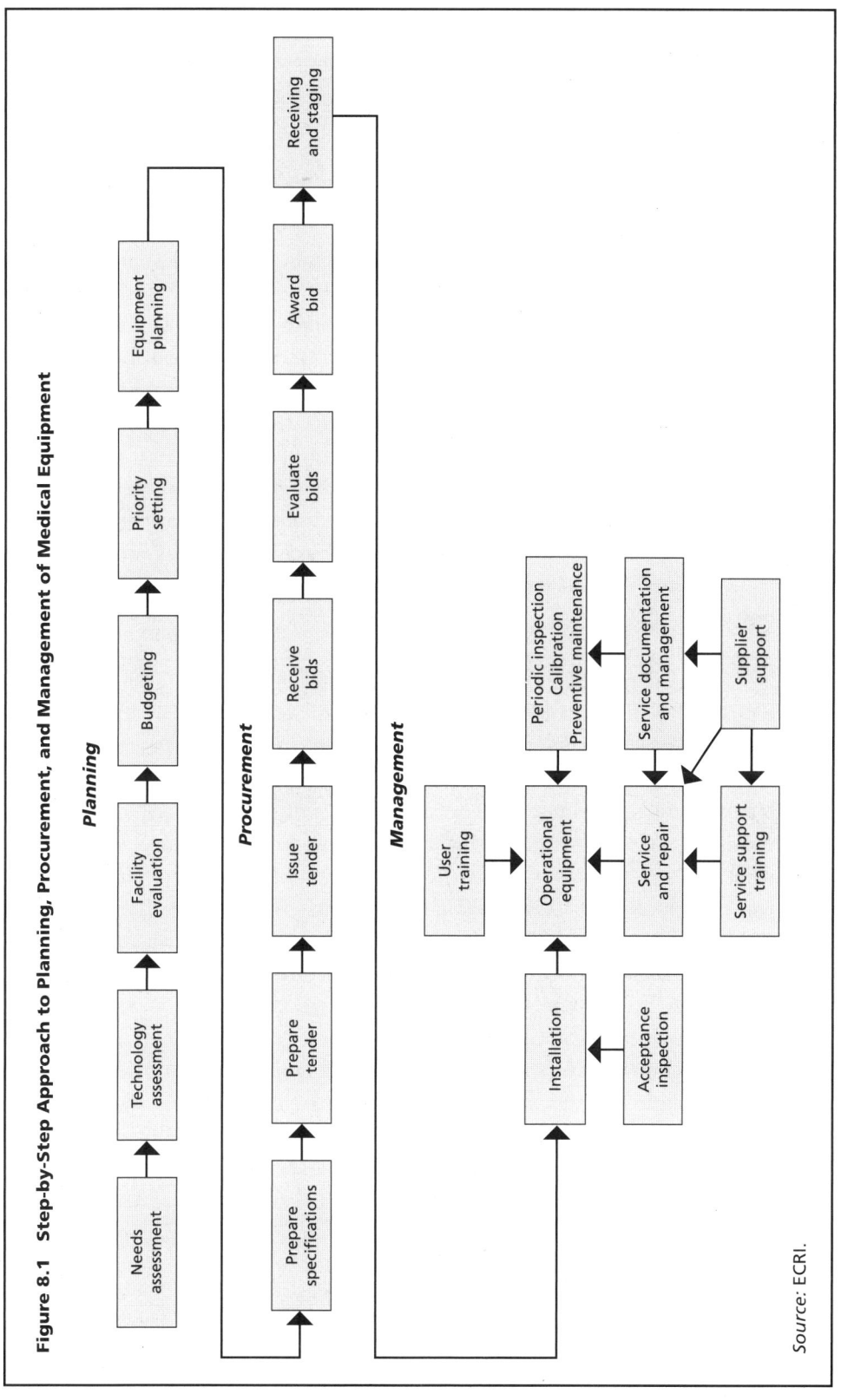

Source: ECRI.

familiarity, the rate of utilization, and an expected rate of return on investment, all of which are discussed further below. Other selection criteria, including safety, are described in appendix P.

Clinical and Technological Adequacy

Many countries require hospitals to have certain essential equipment before they can receive licenses to operate. Therefore, the preparation of equipment and supplies necessary for your hospital's operation should start with the list of essential equipment required by relevant government authorities. In addition, you and your partners may choose to install certain other major medical equipment that you deem critical to perform the functions needed for delivery of the treatments and/or diagnostic procedures planned for your hospital. In analyzing these needs, you should assess any new trends in relevant treatment, diagnostic, or preventive techniques that could become more widely accepted in the following two or three years. Because expensive medical equipment can have a useful life of at least seven to eight years, it is wise to consider whether or not a particular type of equipment or model could handle the expected new techniques.

The rapid pace of technological change in society has meant the faster-than-ever development of new medical equipment. Changes in product materials, data processing, and design have enabled equipment manufacturers to introduce smarter, lighter, and smaller equipment within a shorter time frame than before. It is not wise to purchase a model that is being offered at a very low price because its production is being discontinued. Such equipment risks turning into what industry professionals call "orphan technology," which means that the equipment may not be supported in the future in terms of the availability of supplies, spare parts, and repair and maintenance services. This is mainly a concern with equipment that is more than seven or eight years old, but the circumstances may differ depending on the manufacturer and model.

Similar cautions apply to the question of buying or accepting donations of used equipment. In the case of equipment donated by an institution in a foreign country, details such as adaptability to a different power source and the availability of spare parts and supplies need to be considered carefully before accepting the equipment. For example, a mismatch in the power usage could mean that the equipment would have to rewired or otherwise retrofitted before it can be used. In the event that you have identified suitable used medical equipment, having the equipment's original manufacturer available to refurbish it and certify its functionality will be critically important.

Supplier Reliability

In all cases, it is important to confirm the reliability of the equipment manufacturer. If you are considering a manufacturer whose name is not well known internationally, you may need to ask for references of hospitals and clinics that have been using the company's equipment.

You may not need to be too concerned with the reliability issue if you are dealing with a globally known equipment manufacturer. However, you should assess the ability of the agent or broker to ensure timely delivery and proper installation of your equipment, as well as postinstallation maintenance. It is important to know that the agent/broker has been in the same business for many years, is financially stable, and will not go out of business within a year or two after supplying your equipment. This will be of particular importance if the manufacturer does not have much experience in supplying to overseas clients, especially those in developing countries.

Constraints

Once the equipment is installed, moving and reinstalling it can be cumbersome and costly. Therefore it is necessary to carefully evaluate and determine where the equipment will fit in the hospital, and specific needs for smooth operation of the equipment should be factored into the hospital's design and construction planning. In addition, you will need to consider such details as the distance required between the equipment and windows, walls, and doors; the location of fixtures; the size and swings of doors; and the potential impact that particular floor and wall covering materials could have on the functioning of the equipment. When assessing space needs, attention should also be paid to the daily flow of people, supplies, and any auxiliary equipment, if applicable, and the comfort and ease with which staff can operate the equipment on a daily basis.

User Familiarity

In some cases, familiarity with key medical equipment plays an important role in the mindset of physicians, nurses, and technicians and can affect their productivity. People sometimes develop a sense of ease with the particular equipment that they are familiar with and prefer to continue using it. If you are planning to recruit physicians and technicians whose daily work will require extensive use of a particular type of equipment, especially in a situation where there is limited choice of trained staff available, it may be helpful for you to find out which type of equipment these physicians and technicians are familiar with before making the final selection of equipment.

Utilization Analysis and Revenue Estimation

The amount of revenues that can be generated from operating each piece of key medical equipment has to be estimated as systematically as possible. In other words, revenue per equipment unit should not be projected based on an annual lump-sum approach that does not have a clear basis. Even though the patient's or physician's decision to use certain tests or treatments will not always depend entirely on the cost of the procedure, prices do influence the level of utilization of some equipment. The utilization analysis, therefore, needs to be conducted under several sets of pricing assumptions so that you will be able to obtain a realistic range of revenues that you can expect from operating the equipment.

This exercise will provide you with an opportunity to think about the price sensitivity of tests and treatments. You will need to consider what level of prices will be considered too high, so that people might start avoiding those tests or treatments. Obviously, if the fees are set low enough, people will be more willing to take the tests or treatments. But if the prices for a particular procedure are too low, even a high level of equipment utilization may not enable the hospital to pay all costs and recover the amount of capital invested in that equipment. In that case, you effectively will be providing social services insofar as the use of this particular equipment is concerned. Such usage might be subsidized by the profits generated by other procedures or operations of the hospital. Whether such a situation is financially sustainable has to be analyzed clearly, and if there is a special reason to adopt a low-pricing policy for a certain time in view of the other potential benefits, then such impact needs to be quantified and monitored carefully.

With regard to pricing assumptions, it is a good idea to combine two sources of information. The first is the information on prices charged by other hospitals, which should have been collected during the feasibility analysis. The second is the cost-based approach, based on costs and usage of a given piece of equipment. You can begin with an estimation of the total itemized costs, including financial charges and depreciation, in annual terms for the first two or three years of the equipment's life. Then you divide the total costs by the estimated total number of uses (that is, procedures) in the same period. This will result in a weighted-average cost per procedure for the equipment for the first two- or three-year period. You will then need to add a target profit margin (a percentage over the average cost) to compute the target price per use. The final step is to compare the cost-based indicative prices per use with the price information you have

Box 8.1   ECRI: Advisory Services on Health Care Technology

ECRI is an independent, not-for-profit organization committed to improving the safety and cost-effectiveness of health care technology and hospital operations. Established in 1968, ECRI provides independent and objective research and assessment of health care technologies to government agencies, hospitals, and health systems worldwide.

With a staff of 300 interdisciplinary professionals, ECRI provides fee-based advisory services associated with planning, procurement, and management of health care technologies, including training. Its services include planning for new hospitals, assessment of equipment costs and budgets, and evaluating price quotations in comparison to market rates. It produces more than 35 publications and databases related to health care technology, health care risk management, and health care environmental management.

In addition to its U.S. headquarters, ECRI has regional offices in Asia Pacific, Europe, and the Middle East. ECRI is a collaborating center of the World Health Organization and has been designated as an evidence-based practice center by the U.S. Department of Health and Human Services.

For more information: ECRI, http://www.ecri.org.

obtained from other hospitals and make adjustments as necessary. In estimating the maximum number of times that the equipment can be operated per day or per month, downtimes due to power supply irregularity, routine maintenance, major national holidays, and other possible causes need to be factored in.

Life-Cycle Cost Analysis

When comparing the cost of different equipment, the manufacturer's price is a major factor, but not the only one that needs to be considered. You will need to estimate the "all-in" or life-cycle cost of the equipment and incorporate it into the analysis of the equipment's financial impact over its estimated lifetime—say, seven or eight years. According to ECRI (box 8.1), the life-cycle cost can be defined as "the total cost of ownership, including product, packaging, transportation, related supplies, installation, training of users and support staff, utilities (power, air conditioning, steam, water, gases) inspection, service, retirement, and the money paid to acquire, use, and support the technology."

The life-cycle cost provides the basis for the calculation of cost per use (CPU) over the useful life of the equipment. CPU is defined as "the life-cycle cost plus salaries, fees, and overhead divided by the number of tests or treatments during that life cycle." The CPU calculation should be the basis for comparison of the true life-cycle cost of each piece of equipment being considered. This is an important point, because some equipment may have a relatively low purchase price but may require use of expensive disposable supplies and spare parts. In that case, the life-cycle cost of that equipment could be much higher than the life-cycle cost of equipment that has a higher purchase price but uses supplies that cost much less.

PRICE OF EQUIPMENT AND COST OF DELIVERY AND INSTALLATION

Following initial discussions with equipment suppliers, agents, or brokers, you will request and receive from some of them firm price quotations on specific equipment. When you receive price quotations, be sure to ask which services related to installation, testing, and staff training are covered by the price and which are not. You must compare the full impact of different pricing terms such as freight-on-board (FOB) and cost, insurance, and freight (CIF). Sometimes equipment that appears to cost more to purchase may turn out to be a better value because the supplier's price includes aspects of delivery and installation that would cost you much more if you had to purchase those services separately. It will be necessary to prepare a list of all services needed from the point of shipment (the manufacturer's factory or warehouse) to delivery at your hospital's site, and indicate who will pay for each service, so that you will be able to estimate a realistic cost of purchase.

SUPPLIES AND SPARE PARTS

The quantity and cost of supplies and spare parts needed for smooth daily operation of the equipment must be assessed. In developing countries, locally made supplies may not be available, so all or a substantial portion of the supplies and spare parts may have to be imported, usually sourced from the equipment supplier. In such cases, the possibility of cost increases due to exchange rate fluctuations has to be factored in. Depending on the country, you may also need to assess the possibility of interruptions in the importation of supplies and spare parts and prepare a backup plan.

UTILITIES

Costs of electricity, water, gas, steam, and so on need to be estimated if they are necessary for operation of the equipment. Such costs can be computed on a monthly basis to account for monthly and seasonal variations, if any, and then added up to obtain annual totals that can be used for calculation of the CPU.

STAFF COST

Salary and benefits of the full-time equipment operator will be a key component of staff cost. In addition, costs associated with regular training, the equipment maintenance staff, if applicable, and the administrative staff, if applicable, will also need to be incorporated in the staff-related costs.

REPAIR AND MAINTENANCE

Expenses expected in connection with repair and maintenance can be estimated with the help of the equipment supplier. You will need to estimate the scope and frequency of repair and maintenance work that will be necessary at least on an annual basis. If such services cannot be obtained locally, you should assess the prospects for the availability of local technicians in the following two or three years. Additional discussions concerning repair and maintenance are provided below.

FINANCING COST

If separate financing is to be obtained for the equipment, such as through leasing or equipment financing, it is a straightforward task to calculate the financing cost related to the equipment. If you plan to purchase the equipment with loans from one or more lenders, you will need to estimate the pro rata weighted-average cost of financing applicable to the equipment.

RETURN ON INVESTMENT ANALYSIS

You will be able to use the estimated annual amounts of revenues and costs to calculate the estimated return on investment, which will demonstrate the financial results of owning and operating the equipment. Determining the level of financial return on the amount of capital that will be invested in medical equipment is a subjective matter; however, you may need to ascertain that the equipment can generate at least 15 percent of internal rate of return on capital over the course of the equipment's estimated seven or eight years of useful life.

Procurement

In many countries, the process of procuring medical equipment often starts with a department or unit making a request for equipment. Specifications are written based on the equipment request, and proposals are invited for submission. Proposals are then evaluated and selected to award the contract. Other countries are increasingly using a new approach that starts with a needs assessment followed by an analysis of data on testing, user experience, vendors, and life-cycle costs. The most suitable technology is selected, followed by negotiation of prices and terms and conditions of the contract.[11]

Buy, Lease, or Share?

You will need to consider whether to buy the equipment or obtain usage rights for a fee through a leasing or sharing agreement. Purchasing equipment has advantages and disadvantages. The advantages include having full control over where to install the equipment, how to operate it, and when to sell or otherwise dispose of it; full entitlement to all revenues that can be generated from operating it; and tax savings from the deduction of depreciation of the purchase cost. The main disadvantage is having to finance the purchase up front. Safeguarding and maintaining the equipment is usually the responsibility of the user, regardless of whether the user owns or rents the equipment. In addition to the buy or lease options, there is a third option, which is to obtain equipment free of charge through donation. However, this has its own costs, namely expenses associated with the process of searching for donated equipment and possibly retrofitting the unit to ensure its operability at your hospital.

In many countries, leasing is a common way of obtaining the rights to use equipment (of many kinds, not just medical equipment) owned by someone else. There are two categories of leasing: operating leasing and capital leasing. The operating lease is essentially a medium- or long-term rental arrangement in which the lessee obtains the rights to use the equipment in exchange for paying a monthly or quarterly lease rental. The lessee, the equipment user, is usually responsible for safeguarding, maintaining, and insuring the equipment. A capital lease is an operating lease with an option for the lessee to buy the equipment at a prenegotiated price at the end of the leasing period. Depending on the credibility and stability of the counterpart, a leasing arrangement may work out well or not so well, as illustrated in box 8.2.

The all-in cost including the financing charge needs to be used when comparing the costs of buying and leasing. When considering a leasing arrangement,

---

11. ECRI, "Healthcare Technology: Equipment Procurement" (PowerPoint presentation, 2002).

Box 8.2   Leasing Medical Equipment: One Hospital's Experience

The management team of an 80-bed, secondary care hospital located in a major city in a southern African country thought that it had a good way to equip the hospital with an up-to-date x-ray machine. Under the leasing agreement, a South African company supplied an x-ray machine, financed the construction of the wing of the hospital where the equipment was installed, and took responsibility for maintaining the equipment after its installation. The hospital became the exclusive user of the equipment and paid lease charges based on revenue from use of the machine. According to the hospital staff, the legal ownership of the room where the equipment was installed, as well as of the equipment itself, was in the name of the South African company.

A few years after the hospital began operation, the South African company went into financial difficulties and could not maintain the equipment properly. At the same time, the company became the subject of legal actions taken by its creditors. This led to a court order that prohibited any action concerning the x-ray machine, as well as the room. The x-ray machine needed repair, but the hospital could not do the repair because of the court order. As a result, the hospital could no longer provide key diagnostic services essential to its operations.

There was no other hospital or a diagnostic center that had an x-ray equipment of similar sophistication in the same city or in any city nearby, so the hospital could not even outsource critical diagnostic services. As a result, the hospital's operations and its financial results were negatively affected by the failure of an agreement that was initially thought to be a great solution to the hospital's financial limitations.

---

you should investigate the full details of the conditions, including currency of lease payments and conditions of cancellation (by either the lessor or the lessee), which may include a cancellation penalty. When considering leasing, you will also need to understand each option's implications for accounting and financial reporting and its impact on the calculation of various financial ratios. Signing a lease agreement denominated in foreign currency will have the same effect as taking out a foreign currency loan in terms of foreign currency risk for your hospital. Therefore, you will need to examine your hospital's ability to generate foreign currency earnings before taking on any responsibility for payments that will be denominated in foreign currency.

Another way to obtain use of equipment without buying it is through an equipment-sharing agreement. You might identify an underutilized machine available at an area hospital and rent it on a part-time basis from them. This may be economical, but such an arrangement does entail some risks. These include the possibility that the equipment might suddenly become unavailable for your hospital's use because of a sudden surge in the other hospital's patient flow or some other reason. Even if you write a careful agreement that seems to cover all possible situations, it may not be sufficient. There is always a risk that the other hospital may not abide by the agreement in the course of pursuing its own operational and financial objectives.

On the other hand, if there is a need for an expensive piece of medical equipment in the area but your feasibility analysis shows that your hospital alone would not be able to make full use of it, you might consider buying the equipment and renting it out to other hospitals. This is a more difficult decision to make, because you will be financing the up-front cost of purchase. If your agreement does not specify a guaranteed level of usage of the equipment and the fee associated with such usage on either a monthly or quarterly basis, you run the risk of not being able to generate the expected amount of revenues from such an arrangement. It is also possible that the other hospital may suddenly decide not to use your equipment for one reason or another unless the agreement contains specific conditions in that regard. And even if the counterpart hospital sends the expected number of patients, thus fulfilling the minimum usage requirement, there is the risk that it may not pay the agreed fees in time.

Therefore, an equipment-sharing arrangement has to be carefully considered and should be discussed thoroughly with an experienced lawyer before an agreement is prepared. In addition to the minimum guaranteed amount of fees (essentially a use-or-pay condition), the agreement will need to include the payment method (direct pay by patients is the best approach), provisions for free-of-charge services if applicable, advance notice requirements in the event of equipment repair and maintenance, handling of patient information if applicable, indemnities if applicable, and other details. Negotiating a detailed equipment-sharing agreement, and enforcing such an agreement later on, may be more difficult with a public hospital than with a private hospital.

Evaluation of Bids

If a competitive bidding process is involved, you will need to evaluate the bids. The use of a template response format eliminates bias from the bid evaluation process and gives the buyer a solid basis for comparison of bids. It is essential to carefully evaluate manufacturers' bid responses for completeness and appropriateness.

Purchase Contract

The purchase contract needs to contain most of the following items (in no particular order):

- Specifications of equipment
- Terms of delivery (including port of landing if the equipment is imported, responsibility for customs clearance, and local transportation between the port and the hospital)
- Terms of installation services
- Responsibility for specific actions to be taken by the equipment supplier and the buyer
- Postinstallation testing
- Warranties and indemnities
- Insurance
- Repairs and maintenance services to be provided by the manufacturer
- Supplies to be provided by the manufacturer, if applicable
- Training services to be provided by the manufacturer
- A timetable that will cover every step necessary from the date of signing of the agreement until the day that you issue a written confirmation of the acceptance of the equipment and the installation
- Prices and fees
- Which services will be provided free of charge and which will be charged separately
- Payment terms
- Penalty for delays in delivery and installation
- Escrow account conditions
- Cancellation conditions
- Terms of refund in the event of cancellation
- Any other terms and conditions applicable to your project

It is important to ensure that the equipment purchase agreement is made with the equipment manufacturer directly and not with an agent or a broker, to the extent that local laws allow this. The manufacturer will provide the equipment and services relating to delivery and installation, as well as maintenance and repair. If the manufacturer is not a party to the purchase agreement, it will not have direct contractual responsibility to you to provide the equipment and services. There may be situations in which the services of an agent or broker are needed. In this case a separate agreement with the agent or broker can be prepared, in addition to the agreement with the manufacturer, to describe the scope of services to be provided by the agent or broker, fees, payment terms, and other conditions. If local business laws require local agency representation, you may consider having the equipment manufacturer become the secondary obligator to the agreement that will be signed between the hospital and the agent. It is customary for the buyer to hold a small portion of the payment (about 5 percent) to the equipment supplier in an escrow account until all work related to delivery and installation is completed satisfactorily. The escrow money is paid when the final inspection certification is issued, normally after the installation and test runs of two or three months.

Delivery and Installation

Equipment delivery should be carefully planned to ensure timely delivery and no damage to the equipment during shipment. Depending on the size and complexity of the item, it may take months to receive the medical equipment you have ordered, particularly if the equipment is manufactured in a foreign country. Even when the equipment is made locally, delivery usually takes up to 30 days or even longer. Delivery of medical equipment entails preshipment inspection, proper packaging, documentation of purchase contract and the bill of lading, customs clearance and forwarding of equipment at the landing port, and inspection upon delivery at the hospital. The equipment then must be installed and tested. The entire delivery and installation process when it proceeds normally can take from three to nine months, depending on the country and location of the equipment manufacturer and the hospital.

Any problem that causes unexpected delay in delivery and installation of the equipment can seriously delay your overall building project. Common pitfalls include delays in transit, inaccurate labeling and documentation that holds up customs clearance at the port of entry, and malfunctioning of the equipment resulting from improper packaging (box 8.3). Some buyers choose a low-cost shipping option and experience delays that may cost more than the savings in the shipping cost. Also, damage to equipment during delivery may mean that the equipment has to be shipped back to the manufacturer and the whole process repeated. It is the responsibility of the seller or supplier to prepare all necessary paperwork (for example, the bill of lading, corresponding voucher, and proof of insurance) to ensure smooth clearance through customs. As a buyer, you need to ensure that the party who will handle the delivery process is familiar with all the details relating to it and has the proper manpower to make sure that your equipment is delivered on time and undamaged.

It is important to discuss the exact delivery destination with the equipment supplier. Often, the destination is defined in the procurement documents as the port of entry and not the health care facility itself. When delivery is taken at the port, you as the purchaser may incur unplanned costs to transport the equipment from the port to your facility.

The usual process of installation involves pretesting the equipment before shipping and at the destination before installation, as well as postinstallation testing for proper functioning. Inspection certificates need to be obtained for each of these steps. Because equipment delivery and installation meets several critical milestones of the overall project, the process calls for proper coordination

---

Box 8.3 Faulty Packaging Delays Delivery

As construction of the new Franco-Vietnamese Hospital in Ho Chi Minh City, Vietnam, neared completion, hospital management completed the purchase order of key medical equipment, most of which was imported. The managers thought they had arranged all the details of the shipment and installation and expected no delays in taking delivery. They were therefore alarmed when the equipment's arrival was in fact delayed. Upon inquiring with various parties, they learned that the container in which the hospital's equipment was loaded had been turned away at the Vietnam port of entry and sent back to Singapore.

The reason, it turned out, was that the equipment supplier had combined the Franco-Vietnamese Hospital's equipment with another buyer's equipment in one package for loading. When the container arrived in Ho Chi Minh City, customs officials refused to clear the package because there was more than one bill of lading for one package of goods. The entire package was sent back to Singapore to have the goods repacked in separate packages for each buyer. This caused almost one month's delay for shipping to and from Singapore, and extra cost.

---

among the construction manager, the equipment supplier, the customs clearing agent, if applicable, and the trainer. The construction manager determines the desired timing of the delivery and installation, which is in turn communicated to the supplier.

Manufacturers often deliver and install equipment through specialized third-party companies, and it is recommended that you discuss the availability of such third-party providers with the manufacturers. Such companies are experienced not only in the transport and installation of the equipment but also in the different shipping procedures around the world, including customs requirements.

Training

Your staff must be trained in use of the new equipment. Along with the installation services, manufacturers usually provide a certain level of training free of charge (that is, included in the equipment price). You will need to assess the adequacy of such training and determine whether you need to obtain additional training services for a fee from the equipment manufacturer or its agent to ensure smooth operation of the equipment. Training provided during the preopening stage and for a certain period after the hospital's opening should be regarded as "training the trainer," so that the staff who receives the training from the equipment manufacturer at that time will be able to train others later.

Most imported equipment comes with manuals written in English, German, Japanese, French, or other major languages. If your country does not have many technicians who speak those languages, you may need to have the vendor to provide you with at least key parts of the manuals translated into the local language well before the hospital's opening. This is a challenging task, as equipment manuals usually include much specialized terminology and a poor translation could create problems. Having the vendor provide the translation will not only help ensure the quality of the translation but also avoid any potential copyright violation.

Maintenance and Insurance

Good maintenance increases the productivity and lifespan of any equipment, while the lack of maintenance can cause service interruption, loss of revenues, and damage to the hospital's image. It is extremely important that biomedical technicians knowledgeable about the purchased equipment be available in the country. However, in many developing countries such technicians are in short supply, and many hospitals and clinics thus have to rely on visiting foreign technicians. They may visit some countries only infrequently and may not be available when you need them. Therefore, it is wise to have a backup plan so you will not have to wait for months to get your critical equipment repaired. One possible backup plan is to share technicians who work at other hospitals. Some hospitals have solved this problem by setting up an equipment maintenance company and by obtaining the local franchise of the international companies, sending staff abroad to build the required capacity.

The spare parts inventory needs to be managed in a systematic way so as to ensure an adequate inventory and prevent unnecessary loss of parts due to poor storage or theft. You may want to make a systematic search for lower-cost replacements, including locally produced parts.

ECRI estimates that a health care facility with well-managed systems usually incurs an annual cost of 5–6 percent of the purchase price of the equipment for comprehensive repair and maintenance service. Internally managed radiographic and laboratory equipment services cost annually an average 7–9 percent of the equipment purchase price. The annual cost of comprehensive service including parts, labor, and software upgrades for complex equipment maintained by the supplier is in the range of 10–15 percent of the equipment purchase price, depending on uptime guarantees.

9

Facility Construction

As Planned, on Time, and on Budget

Although construction is an integral component of your hospital project, it is a project of its own with a definite beginning and end. As with any construction project, building a health care facility entails defining the scope of construction, planning the construction, and implementing the plans. However, the building of health care facilities has peculiar aspects because of the special nature and complexity of health care services. It therefore requires special care and preparations.

Along with obtaining financing, building the facility will be one of the most challenging components of your entire project because of the vast array of resources, people, machinery, money, and activities that are involved. It is important to make sure that construction planning is done comprehensively and that the construction process itself, once started, is undertaken according to the plans.

Planning for Construction

The key objective of the planning stage is to ensure that the hospital will be built in accordance with the architectural design that has been selected and that this will be accomplished within the budget (more accurately, within the amount of financing available) and the target timetable. You will most likely move into the construction stage once the following events have occurred or are occurring:

- The outcome of the feasibility analysis has confirmed the project's physical, operational, environmental, and financial viability.
- A construction site of the size and character required for your hospital has been secured. If applicable, fences around the border of the land would have been installed as well.
- A construction manager (preferably a company, not an individual) has been identified and retained.
- The final versions of the design concept and schematic drawings described in chapter 7 have been chosen by you and your partners after full discussions with the core team.
- Detailed cost estimates have been reviewed and discussed fully and a consensus has been reached among you and your partners about the reasonableness of the estimates and the possibility of funding.
- Firm, written commitments of financing have been obtained from credible financial partners (equity investors and lenders) and cover at least 80–90 percent of the total amount of estimated funding needed, including the amount for contingency.
- At least 50 percent of total cash spending needed in the next 12–18 months is available in cash in a bank account, excluding the amount of soft costs that have already been spent.

Documents Needed

By the time the planning of construction begins, various documents should be in hand. These include, first of all, land-related documents: maps, copies of land ownership documents, documents relating to zoning, a site inspection report, a geotechnical test report, and reports on environmental issues and liability assessment. Also needed are agreements relating to the purchase or lease of the land, either the full-scope purchase or lease agreement or a conditional/provisional agreement for land purchase or lease, or a land purchase option agreement.

Second, relevant licenses and permits for construction and construction-related activities must be obtained. For example, if it is necessary to build or pave an access road from the main road to the hospital site, or if a permit is required for movement of construction materials over certain roads or bridges, such permits should be in place before any money is spent for construction work.

Third, the architect's documents should be in hand. These include revised and finalized schematic design drawings, including space program and conceptual design, and conceptual design drawings for one or two alternative options, if necessary. You also need a final contract with the architect that specifies all services required from the architect until completion of construction and testing of the facility's functionality. These may include, among other services, preparation of other construction-related drawings and documents or assistance in the selection of interior design, furniture and fixtures, and so on.

Finally, you will need a list of major medical equipment planned for installation (see chapter 8).

The Construction Team

Parsons META, a U.S.-based professional consultancy firm (box 9.1), suggests that the following specialists or firms are necessary for building a health care facility:[12]

- Architect
- Civil engineer
- Structural engineer
- Mechanical engineer
- Electrical engineer
- Medical communications planner
- Medical information system planner
- Medical equipment planner
- Interior designer
- Landscape architect
- General contractor/construction manager
- Electrical contractor
- Mechanical contractor
- Signage consultant
- Shielding consultant
- Food service consultant
- Surveyor
- Geotechnical consultant

As noted in chapter 7, many of the engineers and specialists listed above are needed during the hospital's conceptual design stage, so it is likely that some of them will already have been identified by this time. Therefore, depending on how you assign major construction components (see the section below on construction assignment), the general contractor you hire before the construction planning stage may be able to provide expertise in many of the areas listed above.

---

12. Parsons META, "Healthcare Design & Construction Checklist," http://www.meta-usa.com/checklist.html.

Box 9.1   Parsons META: Advisory Services on Development of Health Care Facilities

Parsons Healthcare Division, formerly known as META Associates, specializes in managing the planning, design, and construction of health care facilities from inception to completion, acting as the project owners' representative. Its fee-based comprehensive program management services include project management, facility/master planning, engineering/facility condition assessments, conceptual design, medical equipment planning, communications and information technology planning, construction management, interior design, and cost accounting. Headquartered in the United States, Parsons offers its clients free access to its Web-based project management and reporting tool. This tool serves as a platform for team members to schedule and track project deliverables, activities, deadlines, and milestones reached during the life cycle of each project.

For more information: Parsons META, http://www.meta-usa.com.

Construction Management

The construction manager can assist you in estimating construction costs in detail (see appendix Q). Beyond that, the construction manager's role is to help you make decisions on the facility design and construction, to help minimize costs to the extent possible (box 9.2), and to protect your interests by ensuring the high quality of work and services done by various parties. Because of the nature of the job, construction managers are usually compensated with both a monthly retainer and a success fee payable upon completion, as discussed in chapter 4.

The construction manager will take the lead and assist you and your partners, in close coordination with the architect, in finalizing the hospital's conceptual design and the schematic design, developing the construction plan, evaluating various construction techniques available in the area, and estimating costs for construction and other items such as medical equipment. The construction manager will also play the lead role in preparing tender documents in consultation with the lawyer, managing the tender process, evaluating bids received from contractors, negotiating with contractors if applicable, and monitoring the overall daily progress and quality of the contractors' work.[13]

In many developing countries, construction management is a relatively new concept and few if any such firms are available. If it proves difficult to identify a firm that can be retained as construction manager, you may be able to find an individual with substantial experience who can play that role. If the second option is not possible, you may have to approach a general contractor, that is, a construction company, that is well known in the locality and ask it to play the role of construction manager. It will not be an easy task for the general

---

13. Parsons META, "Healthcare Design & Construction Checklist."

> **Box 9.2 Saving on Costs through Construction Management**
>
> A group of physician-entrepreneurs in an African country solicited the services of an architect, a civil engineer, and other building engineering and construction professionals for their new hospital project. They realized that the professional fees of the individual experts would triple their budget stipulation. After rethinking the issue, the physician group decided to hire a construction management company known for managing previous hospital projects in a neighboring country. The construction management firm had its own architects and engineers, and during the actual construction it recruited workers from the city center on a pay-per-work basis. By using the firm, the physicians were able to contain costs within 85 percent of the construction budget. The project also made a substantial local economic impact through the steady employment of local laborers.

contractor, however, as most construction companies, especially those in developing countries, will not have played the role of monitoring their competitors. Whether such a person or firm is called a construction manager or not, an important consideration in getting expert help is to ensure that the adviser has considerable experience in constructing health care facilities.

Construction Risk Assessment

During the construction planning stage, the construction team needs to assess various risks associated with construction and determine how each will be handled. C-Risk, a consulting firm, classifies risks and exposures associated with construction into five main groups: contractual, operational, organizational, financial, and insurable.[14]

Construction planning should also address the routing of construction traffic, hours for construction, access to utilities, safety of construction workers and other staff, safeguarding of construction materials at the site, phases of the construction process, and contingency plans for bad weather or other natural events. If you are expanding or refurbishing an already operational hospital, the construction plan should also detail the measures that will be taken to minimize operational disruption and noise disturbance and maximize infection control during this time. The project's consumption of energy and impact on the environment during the construction stage need to be considered. With increasing environmental awareness and innovations in materials and construction techniques, there are growing efforts for the "greening" of health care facilities. A sustainable approach to construction leads to reduced resource use, reduced disturbance of the site and surrounding areas, and lower costs. Attention to

14. C-Risk, "Risks & Exposures," http://www.c-risk.com/Construction_Risk/CR_Exposures_01.htm.

environmental issues during construction also leads to a safer, healthier working environment for staff involved in all aspects of the construction work, as well as for those who will later occupy and use the facilities.

Documents to Be Prepared during Construction Planning

As the full construction team is being assembled, including the construction manager, a number of key documents need to be prepared.[15] This should be done well before the actual construction begins. The following list of required documents is not exhaustive and will need to be adjusted for your project, but the basic items include:

- The design development documents, which will include all details of the final versions of the architectural plans and drawings, as noted in chapter 7 and described in more detail below
- A list of all medical equipment planned for installation, as described in chapter 8
- A package of documents that will be prepared based on the design development documents and that will be used for the bidding of various construction contracts (the "construction documentation")
- A detailed timetable that identifies all tasks to be completed and that will need to be incorporated into the construction documentation and later into the construction contracts
- A task manager assignment list that shows who will take the primary responsibility in coordinating and monitoring the quality and timeliness of the work to be done

The design development documents will include, among other things, drawings on land elevation; details of the structural, electrical and mechanical aspects of the facility; heating, ventilation, and air-conditioning; communication systems; installation of medical equipment; and the information and technology systems. The design specifications should be as detailed as possible so as to minimize risks associated with misunderstandings about such matters as selection of construction materials and sizes of doors and corridors, as well as the sequence of the tasks to be completed. In addition, the design development documents need to include a room-by-room list of all equipment needed, with detailed specifications for every piece of equipment, as well as details on interior design matters such as room furnishings, surface finishes, materials to be used, and other hardware needed for furnishing of each room.

---

15. This section draws on, among other sources, Dr. Joel Nobel, "Investor Briefing: Health Facility Planning & Development," and Parsons META, "Healthcare Design & Construction Checklist."

Construction companies interested in bidding on construction contracts will use the construction documentation to understand the scope of work needed and materials required, assess their ability to deliver, estimate their bid amount, and prepare their tender documents. Therefore, if the design development documents are not prepared accurately and in sufficient detail, it will affect the contractor's cost estimates in the form of less exact costing. There may also be a higher percentage or amount of cost contingency or profit component to compensate for the uncertainties associated with vague construction requirements.

Construction Assignment

In some countries, particularly those where professional construction managers are readily available, various contractors are selected and hired based on their specialties. The construction manager, in close coordination with the project developer and the architect, manages the work process and timetable and monitors the progress being made by each contractor. In such an environment, a lead contractor may be hired at an early stage of construction planning to build a large portion of the facilities. The lead contractor will participate in the discussions at the construction planning stage and provide advice to the project developer and the architect. The lead contractor will also assist in inviting and evaluating bids from various subcontractors who will take the responsibility for their own specialty areas.

Alternatively, you may consider tendering a bid to a general contractor through a competitive bidding process. This option may be more feasible in certain countries, depending on the local business environment and the general practices of the local construction industry. The general contractor will undertake most of the construction work for a fixed price, although it may subcontract out certain parts of the work. If this option is chosen, it will likely reduce the number of contractors you and your construction manager have to manage. While you will still need to be fully aware of the qualifications of subcontractors and may to some extent need to approve their selection, the general contractor will take the ultimate responsibility for selecting, monitoring, and paying subcontractors. This option can also provide you with better control over the total construction cost because you will be able to transfer cost increase risks to the general contractor under a fixed-price contract.

Unless there is a special reason for not doing so, all contracts should be awarded through a competitive bidding process. The competitive bidding process is highly recommended for hiring of the general contractor (by you and your partners) or hiring of subcontractors (by the general contractor), as discussed above. Detailed procedural guidelines for international competitive bidding are available on the World Bank Web site (see appendix R).

Contract tendering can be done in large categories, which will award most of the work to one or two contractors, or in multiple components, which could be awarded to several contractors. The bidding documents may include a construction contract for the winning contractor to sign, without negotiations or modifications, at the end of the bidding process. The bidding documents can be made available for a fee, which if set high enough will help verify the seriousness of potential bidders and recover part of the cost of preparing various documents.

Structure of Bidding Prices

There are two ways to structure bidding prices: the cost-plus fee and the guaranteed maximum price.

Under cost-plus pricing, the contractor is required to state how much the construction will cost, the rationale for the estimated cost, and the proposed amount of profit that the contractor wishes to earn for the work. The profit may be expressed in terms of a percentage of the total construction cost or a fixed sum. The fixed-sum profit approach will be more beneficial to you because you can control costs better than with the percentage approach. Under the percentage approach, the contractor may be able to increase profits if there is any cost overrun. Therefore, the contractor will have more incentive to control costs under the fixed-sum profit approach.

Under the guaranteed maximum price arrangement, the contractor is required to submit a bid that guarantees a ceiling price for the project. This implies that any costs over and above the guaranteed price will be the responsibility of the contractor. Guaranteed maximum pricing is more advantageous to the project developer/owner than cost-plus pricing. The contractor will be willing to accept guaranteed maximum pricing only if it sees no major risk that cannot be mitigated and/or eliminated by the contractor. If, for example, there is a possibility that the entire construction project may have to be put on hold because a certain permit or license is not obtained by a certain date, and obtaining the license or permit is not the contractor's responsibility, the contractor would not be willing to accept the guaranteed maximum pricing arrangement.

Construction Documentation and Construction Contract

The design development documents will be elaborated further to include specifications for virtually every aspect of the hospital's construction, including materials. These documents will then become construction documentation. The tender documents will include the predrafted construction contracts and the construction documentation (or parts of it, depending on the scope of work that will be tendered), which must be attached to the construction contracts. The construction contracts should be prepared with the help of a lawyer experienced in construction projects. They should include, among other provisions:

- Scope of services and tasks to be completed
- Construction specifications
- Deadlines and milestones
- Provisions for possible modifications to the construction details and/or deadlines
- Composition of the project team to be assigned by the contractor
- Work hours
- Worker safety and environmental protection measures
- Security of the site and materials
- Reasons for delays allowed (typically natural events such as persistent bad weather, earthquake, or flood, and sometimes labor stoppages such as a transportation strike)
- Performance standards
- Insurance requirements for construction performance, worker health and safety, and other matters
- Inspection conditions and conditions for issuance of the acceptance of the facility
- Indemnity of the project developer (you) in the event of any accidents
- Reporting requirements
- Progress billing and payment conditions
- Conditions under which payments can be delayed
- Cancellation conditions
- Any other special conditions

A very important aspect of the construction contract is the performance guarantee. In many developing countries, construction companies operate with limited amounts of capital because construction is a service business, not an asset-based business. Their cash flows tend to fluctuate depending on the timing of their cash receipts for the construction contracts they work on. If a construction company encounters delays in getting paid for the work they have done on one project, the disruption of their cash flow may have negative repercussions for other projects they have underway. Construction companies often have to spend more money than the initial down payments they receive to keep a construction project going. Yet many construction companies, especially in developing companies, may not practice risk analysis and are not experienced in cash flow management. As a result, some get into serious financial trouble even while they are working on a large construction contract, and this can jeopardize completion of the project. In order to manage this risk in a satisfactory manner, you need to require all contractors (to the extent possible) to submit a performance bond or a performance guarantee.

Many countries have surety and performance bond agencies that sell such bonds. If performance bonds are not available, the contractors should be required to submit a performance guarantee issued by credible banks. The performance guarantee should be written in such a way as to give you full control over the withdrawal of funds in case the contractor defaults on its work after having been paid by you, and/or causes any financial damage to you due to delays or other reasons. You will need to conduct research on this matter at an early stage of planning. In the event that your potential contractors cannot obtain either performance bonds or guarantees on terms and conditions acceptable to you, you will need to structure the construction contract and payment conditions in such a way as to ensure that you pay only for the work that has been completed, minimizing any financial risk that you might take on account of the contractor.

The construction contracts usually require that a portion (typically 5 percent) of the contract amount be withheld until all tests and inspections of the completed work are performed to the full satisfaction of the client. The time between the physical completion of the construction and the payment of the final escrow account money is usually about three months.

Insurance Requirements

In order to cover various risks associated with the construction process, you will need to have adequate insurance policies. These may be procured by you or by the contractor. Examples of the risks that require consideration include construction completion (if performance bonds or guarantees are not available); builders' liability (including construction accidents); fire, flood, and earthquake, if applicable, at the construction site; workers' compensation (medical care insurance); and operation of heavy construction equipment and vehicles.

You will need to consult insurance specialists to understand the type of coverage that may be needed and the prices for various insurance policies. It is a good idea to discuss these matters with someone other than an insurance broker and/or agent who may be selling the insurance policy to you so that you can obtain an objective assessment of various types of coverage needed for your project and the most cost-efficient way to structure the insurance policy.

Time to Break Ground

Once all the construction preparations have been completed, the team should undertake a comprehensive review of them, using checklists, before the groundbreaking. While the construction work is underway, careful and close monitoring of progress being made on a daily basis will be critical to successful completion of the project. A list of pitfalls related to construction of health care facilities is shown in appendix S.

As the construction work progresses, you will be busy with a wide array of other tasks in preparation for the facility opening. Key among these is recruitment of medical, nursing, administrative, and other staff, which is discussed further in chapter 10.

The construction phase is not complete until the building commissioning is done. Commissioning is the assessment and management of specific critical functions in order to transform a building into a fully functional facility that is ready for occupancy and use. To that end, commissioning entails a thorough and systematic process of ensuring that building systems and equipment perform according to the final design specifications and that they all work together interactively without any problems. The commissioning stage will also identify any defects that require rectification. Additional discussions on building commissioning, testing, and dry runs are provided in chapter 10.

10

Facility Opening

Preparing for the Big Day

The start of construction marks the time to begin preparing for the opening of your hospital. Depending on the size and complexity of the hospital's physical settings, the construction process itself can take anywhere from 18 months to two years. As the construction work progresses, various other tasks need to be done: scheduling the delivery of equipment, hiring and training staff, preparing for the IT systems, and writing policies and manuals, among others. The construction period is followed by building commissioning and the dry-run period, which together can take at least three to four months.

The period of preopening preparations is almost always hectic. Therefore, every step needs to be carefully planned. In order to assist your team in this process, you may need several sets of planning charts or diagrams. A master action chart will provide an overall picture of key actions and critical time paths. It could, for example, show major groups of actions needed for your hospital's completion, with symbols or other ways of indicating the relationships between different groups of actions or key steps that must occur before other steps can be taken. The master chart should be augmented by several flow charts, one for each major category of action that appears in the master chart. The flow charts are more detailed in terms of specific actions and the persons responsible for performing or coordinating each action. Each flow chart should include a weekly time line.

The key areas discussed below are not presented in any particular sequence. All the actions are critically important to the smooth opening of the hospital and thus need to be carefully planned and monitored as they progress. Such planning and coordinating work has to be tailored to the specific needs of your hospital project.

Staffing

Hiring the right people at the right time will be a key to successful management of the entire process. Salaries and benefits for quality staff will eventually be a large part of your operating budget. However, the additional cost of hiring key people during the planning and preopening stages—rather than later, after opening—will represent a relatively small proportion of your total project cost. These people will have to be hired eventually, and bringing them on board sooner rather than later is a wise investment.

By the time the hospital's construction begins, a CEO should be in place to manage the entire spectrum of activities concerning the project. As discussed in chapters 4 and 7, the CEO will most likely take over from you the central role of day-to-day project oversight and will provide leadership to the entire team as soon as he or she is on board. In addition, if you can afford it, a full-time CFO should be in place by the time the facility planning and design stage begins. If this is not possible, he or she should come on board at least one year before the hospital's opening, meaning that the position should be filled, at latest, by the time construction begins.

In addition to the CEO and CFO, the medical director or director of clinical operations, the director of human resources management (DHR), and various head nurses should be recruited at least six months before the hospital's planned opening. As discussed in chapter 7, the director of nursing (DON) should have been hired at the time of the facility planning and design. If not, the DON should be on board at least 8 to 10 months before the hospital's planned opening. The DON should take the lead role in selecting and hiring head nurses for each clinical department, especially the head nurse for the operating practice or operating room, before the construction is completed.

The CEO, CFO, director of clinical operations (DCO), DON, and DHR will form the hospital's senior management team and establish the hospital's operating policies, procedures, and guidelines. The management team should be supported by several advisory boards, starting with the medical advisory board. The determination of which boards will be necessary and when they should be formed has to be made in consultation with various key people during the early planning stages.

Every position should be filled on the basis of a formal written job description. The managers must take the time to prepare job descriptions for all of their staff in close coordination with the DHR. The most important ones must be approved personally by the CEO, as they should reflect the vision of the hospital. A sample job description for a director of nursing is provided in appendix T.

In terms of physicians and nurses, you will most likely need to fill only a portion of the total number of planned positions during the early period of the hospital's operation. A core team of physicians and nurses should be in place two or three months before the hospital's scheduled opening date. This core team will undertake the operational rehearsals (the "dry runs") described below and carry out other tasks such as helping the management team complete the writing of operating manuals. In addition, the core team members should receive training that will enable them to do their jobs and also provide training to other physicians and nurses who will come on board later. Once a staff member is hired, his or her salary has to be paid, regardless of the hospital's financial performance. Therefore, you need to prepare the staff recruitment plan carefully and consider its potential impact on your cash balance.

For nonclinical tasks such as accounting, billing, sales and marketing, finance, procurement, and inventory management, you may be able to assign more than one function to a staff member during the initial period of your hospital's operation while the scope and volume of transactions are still relatively low. Additional staff can be hired in step with the growth in the hospital's activities and revenues.

Details of human resource management are beyond the scope of this book. However, the importance of creating a positive work environment cannot be overstated. This effort must be based on a clear understanding of and commitment to your hospital's mission and core principles, teamwork, mutual respect among all staff, and professional and personal development through sharing of knowledge and learning. Assessments of candidates for staff positions at all levels should include each person's willingness and ability to join in your efforts to create such a workplace.

Documentation of Operating Policies and Procedures

For the hospital's smooth operation, various operating policies, procedures, and guidelines must be available in writing. Such documents cover clinical operations, management of human resources, handling of environmental matters (including disposal of medical and nonmedical wastes), and various administrative processes. The written policies and guidelines need to be ready before staff recruitment begins in earnest because they provide the basis for professional management and for staff training. Each department head should prepare operating policies and procedures for review and finalization by the management. Once the policies and procedures are in place, staff should strictly adhere to them.

You can make it easier by obtaining sample operating policies and guidelines from other hospitals operating in the country where your hospital will be located and modifying them to suit your hospital's circumstances. These samples can be complemented with information obtained from various international and national health care–related organizations. If you plan to have expatriate staff, the manuals may need to be translated into more than one language.

You will also need to establish quality standards and quality and risk control mechanisms. From an organizational perspective, at least the following five committees should be established, preferably by the beginning of the hospital's operation: (a) an infection control committee (prevention and control of communicable infections); (b) a deaths analysis committee (very common for emergency rooms and surgical units); (c) a committee of medical ethics (to oversee the entire hospital, including any research conducted within the hospital); (d) a committee of ethics in nursing; and (e) an internal accident prevention committee. In addition to committees, you will need to have the quality standards as well as the quality and risk control mechanisms in writing as a part of the hospital's operating policies and guidelines.

Building Commissioning

After the construction is completed, every aspect of the newly built facility needs to be inspected and tested to confirm conformity to the approved design specifications, structural soundness, and readiness for full and smooth functioning. The inspections and testing usually take two to three months. The contract for the general construction contractor will include various tests as the condition for confirmation that construction has been completed. Special attention needs to be paid to testing the readiness of the following:

- The electrical system
- Utilities (including power generators, if applicable, to be used in case of a blackout)
- Telephone lines and cable and wireless telecommunications connections
- Plumbing and sewerage structures
- Flowed-mechanical and acclimatization systems (for various gases, air-conditioning, and vapors)
- Medical equipment
- Medical gas systems (with outlet-by-outlet testing of type of gas, pressure, and flow rate)
- Signaling system (for both operational and emergency needs)
- Firefighting and fire prevention mechanisms
- Kitchen and laundry facilities

- Medical and nonmedical waste treatment and disposal systems

Every country has various regulations concerning the physical setting of health care facilities. The design and planning of the construction work, as well as testing upon completion, need to ensure that the facility meets national and local regulatory requirements of the country where it is located.

Medical Equipment

As discussed in chapter 8, the installation and testing of major medical equipment will most likely be carried out by the equipment supplier or manufacturer. The precommissioning check of all medical equipment and medical gas systems, however, must be conducted by an independent biomedical engineering firm that is not related to the equipment suppliers and that is properly equipped and staffed for the task. The firm should provide you with a written certificate of functionality verification. Precommissioning inspection of all medical equipment should also include creation of computerized individual equipment records to facilitate lifetime management of inventory, service, costs, and product recalls.

The testing of various equipment, which should be done based on a checklist, normally takes on average two to three months. You will also need to stock supplies critical to the operation of the equipment and define actions to be taken in case of any sudden malfunction or other problems.

IT System

Ideally, the IT system (including the MIS/HIS) should be selected and the relevant contracts put in place by the time the construction begins. This will provide you with sufficient time to manage the process of customizing the system, preparing manuals, purchasing the hardware systems, installing hardware and software, training, and testing the systems before the hospital begins operations. The IT system includes the wireless communication system as well as the personal computers that will be installed for point-of-transaction data entry at various locations within the hospital.

The contract for purchase of the IT system should include details of what the supplier will provide in terms of customizing the system, installing it, testing it, making postinstallation adjustments if necessary after the hospital begins operation, providing periodic upgrades, providing routine maintenance and troubleshooting, providing detailed manuals, and training staff to use the system. The contract should also include specific deadlines for delivery of each component of the system and related services, as well as the procedures for confirmation of your acceptance of the system and services.

The terms of payment of fees for the initial package, as well as for services to be provided afterward, need to be formulated carefully. You do not want the hospital to get into a situation of not having a fully operational IT system after having paid all the fees. You may want to negotiate withholding 5 percent of the total payment in an escrow account until everything has been provided to your full satisfaction. In addition, you may wish to consider and negotiate with the supplier a penalty/bonus component in the payment structure. Under this approach, the buyer and supplier agree on a base price and conditions for installment payments of the base price, related to the delivery of each critical component of the system and services. In addition, a discount or a bonus can apply if the system and services are delivered before the agreed-upon deadline or exceed the required standards of quality. The structuring of the agreement for procurement of the MIS/HIS package is a complicated task that must be done with the help of an experienced lawyer.

The importance of having the manual for the IT system available in the local language cannot be overemphasized. The translation of the manual and checking of the translation for accuracy often take more time than one might expect.

Operating Licenses and Permits

A detailed checklist of various permits and licenses should be prepared with indications of when each one will be needed and who will be responsible for securing it. The licenses and permits will include not only those pertaining to medical practice, emergency care, utilities, waste treatment and disposal, and so on, but also various legal documents necessary for running the hospital as a business.

Obtaining the assistance of a law firm with experience in preparing all paperwork and handling procedural matters concerning permits and licenses can save time and unnecessary frustration.

Minor Equipment and Supplies

A hospital needs a wide variety of smaller equipment as well as medical and nonmedical supplies. Some can be reused multiple times, but many are disposal items for one-time use. Here again, a master checklist of minor equipment and supplies (grouped into reusable and disposable items) should prepared, with in-

---

Box 10.1 Pareto Analysis and Inventory Management

In managing inventory, a good back-of-the-envelope rule is to use what is known as Pareto analysis. This is a method of classifying items according to their relative importance. The first step in the analysis is to identify the usage rate of an item and its unit value. Close control is important for fast-moving items with a high unit value. But for slow-moving, low-unit-value items the cost of the stock control system may exceed the benefits to be gained, and simple methods of control should be substituted.

    The two factors, usage rate and unit value, can be multiplied to obtain the annual requirement value (ARV), which is the total value of the annual usage of each item. When the cumulative ARV is plotted against the number of items, a graph known as a Pareto curve is obtained. The curve will typically show that 80 percent of total ARV is contributed by 20 percent of total number of items. In other words, if a hospital with a stock list of 1,000 different items can manage the top 200 items well, using a sophisticated stock control system, it can control successfully about 80 percent of its total investment in inventories. The next 40 percent of items typically account for a further 15 percent of cumulative ARV. The last 40 percent of items usually consist of low-value and low-volume items and account for about 5 percent of total inventory in terms of value. Such items can be managed with a simple tracking system.

---

dications of when they will be needed for the opening of the hospital, minimum quantities needed, the suppliers, and order schedules.

When preparing the list of supplies, try to purchase the type of supplies with which your clinical staff is most familiar. Physicians and nurses often prefer to use familiar items. Some hospital operators emphasize the power of habit and warn that one should not underestimate the potentially negative impact that new drugs and supplies can have on the productivity of clinical staff, especially if the new supplies are introduced on short notice. Some believe that physicians and nurses may even seek work at a different facility in order to have access to the equipment and supplies that they are accustomed to using.

Careful inventory management can help minimize expenses on minor equipment and supplies. Items of high value and importance should receive more detailed attention than less valuable items (box 10.1).

Insurance

Appropriate insurance policies are essential to cover the numerous risks associated with this period. As noted earlier, you will need to consult an insurance agent or broker (who will not be selling the policies to you) on the types of risks that are relevant to your hospital during the preopening and postopening stages and the pricing available, in the form of either a master policy or separate policies. Typical risks that need to be covered by insurance during this stage include workmen's compensation; medical malpractice; fire, flood, and earthquake, if applicable; and motor vehicles.

The "Hotel Management"

Well-organized, well-equipped, and well-managed auxiliary services are indispensable to the smooth operation of a hospital. The most important of these are food service, laundry, and cleaning. Although nonmedical in nature, they have a large impact on patient satisfaction. It is believed that as high as 90 percent of all complaints received by private hospitals are related to nonclinical "customer service." With the growing speed of information sharing and changing attitudes toward consumer rights, patients and their families are demanding higher standards of comfort. In view of this trend, some private hospitals hire people with experience in hotel management to handle all nonmedical customer services. Provision of high-quality services by caring staff will create a sense of well-being among patients and visitors.

Auxiliary services should be carefully planned in conjunction with clinical services. For food service, a nutritionist needs to be on board to supervise proper preparation and management of patient meals in accordance not only with government regulations but with the standards that you and your management team wish to maintain. In addition to the clinical requirements, you will need to assess the expected growth in volume of food services and ensure that the kitchen layout, equipment, and logistical details are prepared in a way that will support this growth. With regard to cleaning, the installation of equipment should enable janitorial crews to carry out hygienic cleaning of all areas of the hospital without difficulty.

You might wish to consider the possibility of outsourcing such services if there are qualified and experienced contractors available in the area. In analyzing the pros and cons of outsourcing, you should estimate the time and costs involved in hiring and training the staff that would provide these services in-house. These estimates should include provisions for extra space, staff, and equipment to cope with increasing volumes and with emergencies. This should then be compared to the costs—and risks—of contracting out these functions. Factors to consider before making the decision include (a) the all-in cost of each option, (b) the track record and reputation of the potential outside contractor(s), and (c) the operational and financial reliability of the contractor(s). Obviously, you want to avoid the possibility of having services interrupted because the contractor goes bankrupt or has other problems. Potential contractors should be required to provide written documentation of their service records and financial strength, along with references from other clients. You will need to carry out a background check on the contractor, including a search for any complaints filed against the company, before signing a contract. It is wise to have a standby contractor who is ready to step in and provide the services your hospital needs should your primary contractor become unable to deliver the services.

Training and Support System for Troubleshooting

Under the guidance and leadership of the director of human resources, a master plan and timetable for training programs must be prepared. For key medical and nonmedical equipment, the equipment supplier or manufacturer should provide training as a part of the purchase contract. For certain areas, it may be possible for you to arrange training of your staff at one or more nearby hospitals. If possible, you may also consider a swap arrangement where your staff receive training at another hospital before your hospital opens in exchange for training that you would offer their staff in the future. Such an arrangement can save on costs if it can be done in a practical and effective way.

As a part of the training and contingency planning system, you will also need to establish guidelines for actions to be taken in the event of emergency or other unexpected situation. Such situations could concern personnel, the IT system, equipment management, and so forth.

Dry Runs

You and your staff should conduct operational rehearsals or "dry runs" at least two months before the hospital's scheduled opening date. You will need to select a set of three or four different clinical procedures—one or two relatively complex procedures, including an emergency case, and one or two simple procedures—and go through each step of the process, from intake to discharge. The idea is to duplicate the experiences of both patient and staff from the moment the patient enters the hospital until the moment he or she leaves it. Such rehearsals must be comprehensive, covering every step that needs to be taken, including preparation of all documents to be filled out both for patients and for internal filing purposes. The full course of selected procedures should be rehearsed at least three or four times to make sure that no step is forgotten.

At the end of each rehearsal, notes should be taken to identify areas that require improvement. The rehearsals will provide you and your staff with opportunities to remember and follow proper procedures, ensure an adequate stock of supplies, check the security and safety systems, practice mechanical operation of facilities and equipment, and work out measures for the comfort of patients and visitors. In addition, they will allow you to measure the amount of time needed to care for different types of patients. These data can then be used

---

Box 10.2   10 Common Mistakes to Anticipate and Avoid

1. Unrealistic expectations regarding cost, time, and space: budgets that are too lean, schedules that are too tight, and spaces that are too small for the functions they need to accommodate.
2. Failure to allow the necessary lead time for purchased items to be delivered, installed, and tested.
3. Inexperience among project participants relative to the specific type of health care facility or project, or the various design requirements applicable to the geographic area.
4. Changes relating to project design, especially last-minute changes that affect the intent or the scope of the project. These can cause delays in the hospital's opening and revenue generation.
5. Personnel changes during the project that result in deviations from the original operational intent.
6. Unchecked miscommunication and/or misunderstanding of various tasks.
7. Lack of contingency plans for construction-related incidents and other unforeseen problems and emergencies.
8. Hasty opening of the hospital before it is fully ready for operations. Unresolved issues may include inoperability of some equipment, lack of key supplies, problems with the IT system, absence of written operating policies and manuals, and incomplete staff training. Do not assume that deficiencies in the hospital's facilities or staff training can be remedied after opening.
9. Selection of designers and contractors driven by low cost rather than performance value.
10. Poor cash management. Every effort should be made to maintain a sufficient amount of cash in the bank to cover the spending needed for the next six to eight months during the preopening period and the next 12 months—at least—after the hospital's opening.

Source: Adapted from Michigan Department of Consumer and Industry Services, Division of Health Facility and Services, Health Facilities Evaluation Section, Health Care Facility Projects: Project Planning to Opening Survey Recommendations, www.michigan.gov/documents/cis_bhs_fhs_bhs_hfs_554_37376_7.pdf.

---

to make any necessary adjustments in scheduling or staffing for the early period of your hospital's operation.

Hasty opening of a hospital before it is fully ready for operations is a pitfall that must be avoided. Box 10.2 summarizes common mistakes in the overall process of establishing a new hospital, and appendix U offers some helpful "dos and don'ts" for making your project a success.

Opening Day Preparations

As the construction nears completion and the date for the start of operations becomes more certain, you will start planning various events to celebrate the hospital's opening. As discussed in chapter 6, such events are an important marketing tool, as the opening will be one of the best opportunities to gain publicity for the new facility. There are many ways to carry out such events at minimal cost. One idea is to partner with other entities (for example, hospitals, research institutes or programs, equipment manufacturers, pharmaceutical companies, diagnostic laboratories, media companies) with which your hospital is collaborating or will collaborate in the future.

As the big day nears, it is wise to anticipate and prepare for delays and mishaps. Numerous events—political or social upheavals, for example, or bad weather—could delay the hospital's opening or greatly reduce turnout for the opening events. Even if the opening goes forward on the date planned, a VIP who was scheduled to be a keynote speaker at the opening ceremony might suddenly cancel or simply fail to show up.

Also of concern are events that could cause a slower-than-expected pace of growth in the hospital's revenue generation. For example, during the bird flu outbreak in Asia in late 2003 and early 2004, people became reluctant to visit hospitals out of fear of coming into contact either with bird flu patients or with medical personnel who might have had contact with infected patients. At least one new hospital that opened in an affected country experienced significant delays in building up its patient base and revenue generation.

Health-related events are obviously relevant, but non-health-related events may be as well. For example, political events in the country could set off worker strikes or general demonstrations. You will need to closely watch any developing stories at the global, national, regional, and local levels with an eye to the

---

Box 10.3   A Success Story: The Opening of Reddington Hospital

Nigerians were thrilled when a multispecialty health care facility known as Reddington Hospital opened in Lagos in 2006. The country's president offered glowing commendations, describing the newly commissioned hospital as helping to meet the ever-increasing need for tertiary institutions to provide first-class medical services to Nigerians.

Reddington Hospital began operations in 2001 as a small cardiac center in close association with Cromwell Hospital, an established health care provider in the United Kingdom. The primary goal of the cardiac center was to provide comprehensive one-stop care for cardiac-related illnesses.

In just over five years, Reddington was transformed from a single-specialty cardiac center to a multispecialty hospital providing services in cardiology (with coronary and intensive care units), renal dialysis, obstetrics and gynecology, pediatrics, specialized and day-cases, surgeries, ophthalmology, ear-nose-throat, radiology, and psychiatry. It has grown from a one-floor, one-unit center to a nine-floor, multiunit tertiary hospital with 12 outpatient consulting suites, diagnostic and imaging units, adult intensive care unit, coronary care unit, dialysis unit, dental surgery unit, eye clinic, and physiotherapy unit, all within the same premises.

The Reddington Hospital story illustrates a core principle in ensuring success in building health care facilities in developing countries: start small and grow big.

For more information: Reddington Hospital, http://www.reddingtonhospital.com/home.htm.

possible impact on your hospital's opening. To the extent possible, you should prepare contingency plans for coping with such uncertainties.

Establishing a new private hospital in any country is a challenging undertaking. It is even more daunting in the context of a developing country. Yet many private hospitals have been built and operated successfully in the developing world and are making great contributions to their communities and countries (box 10.3). With meticulous and realistic planning and careful execution of every step, coupled with compassion and a strong desire to provide service to others, you too may succeed in opening a brand-new hospital that you and your partners can be proud of—one that will meet critical needs in the community while providing a viable business for you. It is hoped that this book can be a useful tool in making such a worthwhile dream come true.

Appendix A

Sample Timeline for Building a Health Care Facility

This timeline of a typical major project shows the long-range consequences of delays in a sequential undertaking. The timeline is reproduced by permission from *Building a Hospital: A Primer for Administrators*, originally published by the American Hospital Association in 1978. Even though considerable time has passed since the chart's first publication, we feel that most of the steps it illustrates are highly relevant and provide a useful overview of the process covered in this book. Note that the steps leading up to the feasibility analysis, such as concept development and the prefeasibility analysis, are not reflected in the chart.

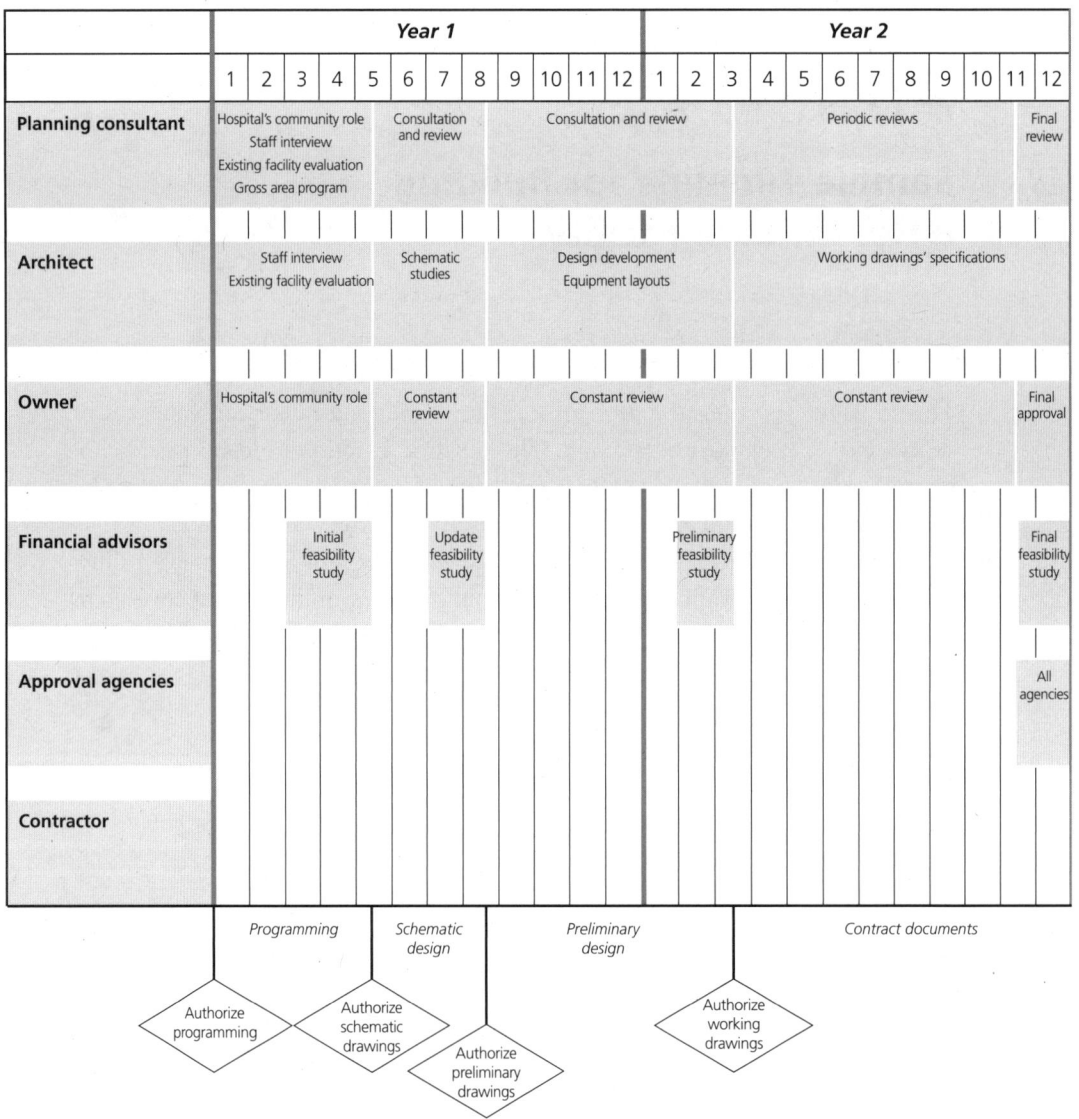

Source: Rea, Frommelt, and MacCoun (1978).

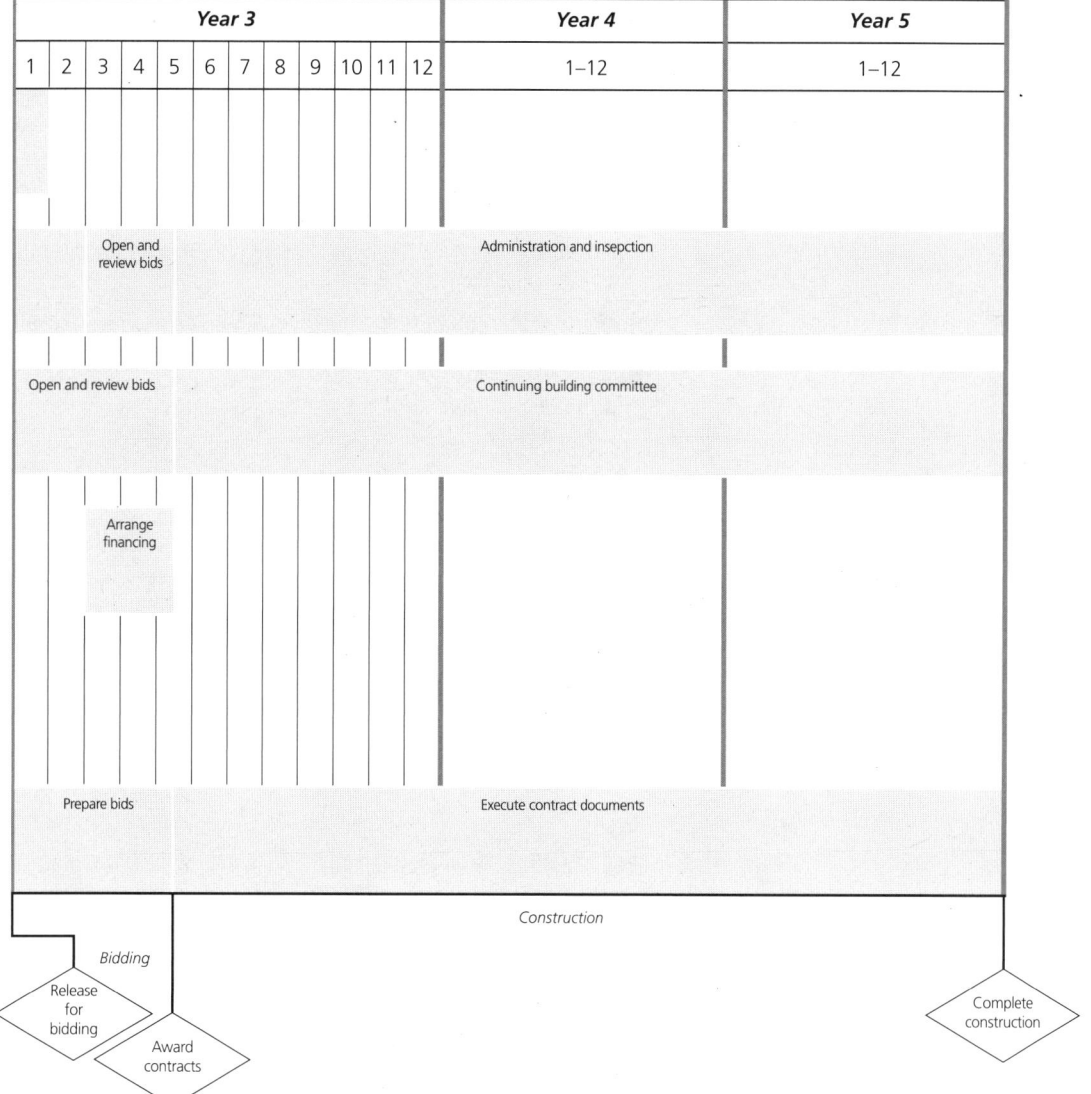

Appendix B
Millennium Development Goals

In September 2000, the United Nations Millennium Summit brought together the largest gathering of world leaders in history. In the summit's final declaration, signed by 189 countries, the international community committed to a specific agenda for reducing global poverty. The goals listed below today guide the efforts of virtually all organizations working in development.

Goal 1. Eradicate extreme poverty and hunger

- Halve, between 1990 and 2015, the proportion of people whose income is less than one dollar a day.
- Halve, between 1990 and 2015, the proportion of people who suffer from hunger.

Goal 2. Achieve universal primary education

- Ensure that, by 2015, children everywhere, boys and girls alike, will be able to complete a full course of primary schooling.

Goal 3. Promote gender equality and empower women

- Eliminate gender disparity in primary and secondary education, preferably by 2005, and to all levels of education no later than 2015.

Goal 4. Reduce child mortality

- Reduce by two-thirds, between 1990 and 2015, the under-five mortality rate.

Goal 5. Improve maternal health

- Reduce by three-quarters, between 1990 and 2015, the maternal mortality ratio.

Goal 6. Combat HIV/AIDS, malaria, and other diseases

- Have halted by 2015 and begun to reverse the spread of HIV/AIDS.
- Have halted by 2015 and begun to reverse the incidence of malaria and other major diseases.

Goal 7. Ensure environmental sustainability

- Integrate the principles of sustainable development into country policies and programs and reverse the losses of environmental resources.
- Halve by 2015 the proportion of people without sustainable access to safe drinking water and basic sanitation.
- Have achieved by 2020 a significant improvement in the lives of at least 100 million slum dwellers.

Goal 8. Develop a Global Partnership for Development

- Develop further an open, rule-based, predictable, nondiscriminatory trading and financial system.
- Address the special needs of the least developed countries.
- Address the special needs of landlocked countries and small-island developing states.
- Deal comprehensively with the debt problems of developing countries through national and international measures in order to make debt sustainable in the long term.
- In cooperation with developing countries, develop and implement strategies for decent and productive work for youth.
- In cooperation with pharmaceutical companies, provide access to affordable essential drugs in developing countries.
- In cooperation with the private sector, make available the benefits of new technologies, especially information and communications.

Source: World Bank.

Appendix C
Types of Public–Private Partnerships

Contract Services

Operations and maintenance. A public partner (federal, state, or local government agency or authority) contracts with a private partner to provide and/or maintain a specific service. Public partner retains ownership and overall management of the public facility or system, for example, laundry, specialized laboratory services, and pharmacy.

Operations, maintenance, and management. A public partner contracts with a private partner to operate, maintain, and manage a facility or system providing a service. Under this contract option, the public partner retains ownership of the public facility or system, but the private party may invest its own capital in the facility or system. For example, the Cambodian government contracted private providers to provide basic health services for districts ranging in population from 100,000 to 180,000.

Lease

Under a long-term leasing arrangement, the private party leases an existing facility from a public agency, invests its own capital to renovate, modernize, and/or expand the facility, and then operates it under a contract with the public agency. This approach could be used in situations where the government does not wish to or cannot, for a variety of reasons, privatize the health care facility and wishes to maintain ownership of the facility. In order to make the investment required for renovation worthwhile, the private party typically asks for a long-term agreement that includes limited conditions under which the lease agreement can be terminated by the public agency.

Build-Operate-Transfer (BOT)

The private partner builds a facility to the specifications agreed to by the public agency, operates the facility for a specified time period under a contract or franchise agreement with the agency, and then transfers the facility to the agency at the end of the specified period of time. For example, the South African government contracted with a private company to build and equip a district hospital. The facility will become government property in 25 years.

Build-Operate-Own (BOO)

The contractor constructs and operates a facility without transferring ownership to the public sector. Legal title to the facility remains in the private sector, and there is no obligation for the public sector to purchase the facility or take title. For example, the state of Victoria in Australia contracted two private organizations to construct a new $56 million regional hospital.

Buy-Build-Operate (BBO)

The government sells an existing facility, which usually requires rehabilitation or expansion, to the private sector entity, which then makes the improvements necessary to operate the facility in a profitable manner. For example, Columbia/HCA, a U.S.-based private hospital company, bought a public hospital for $70 million in Texas that serves a high proportion of low-income residents.

Sources: Tonia Marek, Chiaki Yamamoto, and Jeff Ruster, "Private Health: Policy and Regulatory Options for Private Participation," *Public Policy Journal* 264 (June 2003); U.S. General Accounting Office, *Public-Private Partnerships: Terms Related to Building and Facility Partnerships* (Washington, DC: GAO, 1999).

Appendix D
Health Status Indicators

Following are some examples of health indicators that you may consider obtaining during the prefeasibility study. It is suggested that you try so far as possible to obtain data that reflect your specific geographic target area.

Basic Health Indicators

Population size and distribution by age
Population growth rate
Life expectancy
Crude birth and death rates
Total fertility rate and age-specific fertility rate
Total live births
Female literacy rates

Other Health Indicators

Neonatal mortality rate
Infant mortality rate
Child mortality rate
Maternal mortality rate
Leading causes of mortality by age and sex
Leading causes of morbidity by age and sex
Leading causes of hospitalization by age and sex

Access and Utilization Indicators

% of population with access to medical facilities
Number and geographic distribution of hospitals and residential care
Number of hospital beds per 100,000 population
Hospital bed occupancy rate
Hospital admission rates
Average length of stay in hospital
Average number of physician visits per year
Average number of dental care visits per year

Health Human Resource Indicators

Number and density of physicians
Number and density of nurses and midwives
Number and density of dentists
Number and density of pharmacists

Selected National Health Accounts' Indicators
(at both aggregate and per capita levels)

Total health expenditure
Government health expenditure as % of total health expenditure
Social health insurance expenditure as % of government health expenditure
Donor/external sources for health as % of total health expenditure
Private health expenditure as % of total health expenditure
Out-of-pocket expenditure as % of private health expenditure
Private prepaid plan expenditure as % of private health expenditure

Appendix E

Health Facility and Hospital Development

Joel J. Nobel, MD

Dr. Joel J. Nobel, founder and president emeritus of ECRI, offers the following suggestions based on his long experience in the U.S. and international health care industries. Part I presents a rough time line for development of a health facility, part II examines typical costs for building a hospital, and part III discusses some cost variables.

Part I. Health Facility Development Process Chart

1. Feasibility study (4–6 months)
   - Demographics
   - Epidemiology
   - Clinical needs
   - Market analysis
   - Competition analysis
   - Gap analysis
   - Proposed services
   - Licensing requirements
   - Obstacles
   - Cost projections
   - Projected revenue
   - Profitability projections

2. Decision point
   - Appoint project manager, medical planner, architect, surveyors
   - Institute site search and acquisition and geotechnical studies

- Evaluate special consultants
- Apply for licenses and permits
- Explore financing

3. Project brief (6–8 months)
   - Master plan
   - Architectural concepts
   - Circulation plan
   - Clinical services
   - Preliminary schematics
   - Cost projection

4. Decision point
   - Confirm architectural engagement
   - Engage special consultants (in structural engineering, mechanical/electrical/plumbing engineering, interior design, laboratory design, acoustics engineering, medical equipment planning, laundry and food service, vertical transport, materials management, waste management, central sterile supply room (CSSR), communications, IT, picture archiving and communication system, security and safety systems engineers, and value analysis)
   - Confirm financing arrangements

5. Schematic design phase (4–6 months)
   - Structural design
   - Refine schematic design
   - Preliminary mechanical, electrical, and plumbing design
   - All specialized consultants as required

6. Design development phase (6 months)
   - Architects
   - Specialized consultants as required

7. Contract document phase (6 months)
   - Architects
   - Specialized consultants as required

8. Tendering (2 months)

9. Bid analysis and comparison (1 month)

10. Contract award
  • Management (appoint construction manager)
  • Schedules
  • Safety
  • Quality monitoring

11. Construction phase (12–16 months)
  • Monitor schedule, safety, materials quality, contractor performance
  • Stage delivery and installation of specialized materials and equipment
  • Maintain security

12. Precommissioning phase (2 months)
  • Electrical coordination inspection and testing
  • Medical gas system inspection and testing
  • Medical equipment inspection and testing
  • Obtain occupancy permit

Total project time: 48–60 months.

Part II. What Does It Cost to Develop and Build a Hospital?

The following budget guidelines apply to a nonacademic acute-care general hospital. It assumes the following:

  • The facility will be built on an open site that does not impose challenges in preparation of footings or trenching for utilities.
  • The site will allow a large footprint and at least 4,000 square meters and preferably more per floor.
  • Utilities such as water, sewerage, natural gas, electricity, and telecommunications are adequate and available at the edge of the site.
  • The facility will not include highly specialized clinical units such as burn, cancer, or trauma centers.
  • Outpatient facilities are not disproportionately large.
  • The facility does not exceed four or five floors in height.
  • There is no below-ground garage and no above-ground parking structure.

Given the assumptions above, an approximate breakdown of costs is presented below. Each category of costs is expressed as a percentage of total construction cost.

Element	Percentage of construction costs
Feasibility study	¼ – ½ of 1%
Project brief	½ of 1% – 1%
Architectural and engineering design, specification, and contract documents	8% – 10%
Land	< 20%
Equipment and furnishing	30% – 40%
Precommissioning acceptance inspection of facility and equipment and generation of asset management database	1% – 1½%

For example, a project with $30 million devoted to construction would have fees of $3–$4 million and equipment and furnishing costs of approximately $10–$12 million. However, these rough indices are subject to many qualifications. For example, specialty hospitals, extensive outpatient operations, or small hospitals often require a higher percentage of cost devoted to equipment. A higher percentage of costs for equipment also may apply in nations where costs for construction labor and materials are relatively low. Specialty hospitals may have either more or fewer beds than nonspecialty hospitals.

Total construction costs, excluding land, typically range from $150,000 to well over $300,000 per bed. This range relates to a number of variables such as hospital size and type, choice of materials and finishes, equipment level and sophistication, and specialty clinical services. Furthermore, bed complement, a traditional measure of a hospital, is now far less meaningful as patient length-of-stay is radically reduced and new technology shifts some procedures from inpatient to outpatient. A cost-per-bed projection is therefore less meaningful than it was in the past.

Another construction cost index is cost per square meter, which typically ranges from $2,000 to $3,500 depending on quality of finishes, materials, and hardware.

Part III. Cost Variables with Hospital Development

Regardless of how many hospitals have been constructed, local conditions, choices, and unanticipated circumstances lead to significant cost variations. Using averages drawn from experience can provide a crude index of costs, but specifics dictate the real numbers. Even after construction contracts are awarded inevitable change orders will increase costs. Therefore virtually all development projects have budgeted contingency allowances, typically of 10 percent.

Accurate costs *cannot be determined* before the architectural, interior design, and engineering drawings and specifications are generated, and equipment and furnishings for the facility and patient care are planned on a room-by-room basis and aggregated and priced. This is why it is impossible to provide an equipment list and budget before the architectural schematics and room lists are completed. There are other factors that impact capital requirements. Equipment costs, for example, can be distributed over a future period through leasing or reagent or shared risk per-use contracts.

Some of the other variables that affect costs include:

- Geological and terrain characteristics that impact excavating and foundations costs, sometimes by millions of dollars
- Proximity of adequate electrical, natural gas, potable water, sewage lines, telephone and fiber-optic connections, and roads (the cost of extending utilities to the building can add millions of dollars)
- Parking requirements
- Staff housing requirements
- Type of construction, for example, reinforced concrete versus steel and curtain walls
- Special environmental conditions, for example, special security provisions and controls or water diversion to avoid flooding
- Choice of surface finishes on floors and walls and quality of lighting, doors, and hardware
- Clinical services to be provided, for example, radiation therapy departments can have costs exceeding $8 million for equipment alone
- Incorporation of a hospital information system (most hospitals now incorporate an information system at a typical cost of $2 million to $6 million)
- Incorporation of picture archiving system
- The clinical and administrative quality assurance system to be employed, for example, JCAHO, JCI, or ISO
- Taxes
- Quality of planning (excellent detailed planning minimizes costly change orders to correct errors or the undertaking of important but unplanned work; change orders implemented during construction may range from only 1–2 percent of construction costs to over 20 percent)

Another factor to consider is that the most costly areas, such as imaging, radiation therapy, and clinical pathology laboratories, have similar equipment costs whether the hospital is 100 beds or 200 beds. Therefore the investment in specialized technical infrastructure will be underutilized in the 100-bed facility unless it supports substantial outpatient operations, but the fixed costs are unlikely to change.

Appendix F
Evaluating and Selecting Hospital Consultants

Joel J. Nobel, MD

Evaluating and selecting a consultant is a bit like choosing a spouse. Consider the four Cs: character, capabilities, competence, and chemistry. Except for chemistry, it is very difficult to discern these characteristics accurately during the courtship phase when your intended is on his or her best behavior—and so are you. But here the analogy breaks down, because an experienced consultant has gone through many "marriages," usually for money, but sometimes for love if the project is exciting. You are paying for that experience. Let us explore the first three Cs and outline some of the key questions that you should ask.

Character

Character and values are at least as important as capabilities and competence. What are the central values of the consultant? Explore the consultant's boundaries for potential conflicts of interest. A commitment to technical excellence, objectivity, loyalty to the project, and personal honesty are values you seek and every consultant claims but not all fulfill. Does the consultant simply want to get as much money as possible for doing the job quickly and moving on to another client? How can you discern the difference?

Actions speak louder than words. There is usually little relationship between consulting "cosmetics" such as glossy advertising, beautiful brochures, fancy PowerPoint presentations, glib claims, and even the size of an organization, on the one hand, and its real character and values and how well its consultants will do your job, on the other.

Marketing and promotion of consulting services are typically done by articulate senior consultants, but when the job starts, relatively junior and in-

163

experienced staff members may be assigned to your project. Where are those impressive people who convinced you to sign a contract? Probably out prospecting for other clients rather than leading the team working on your job. Obviously you want to evaluate the individuals who will actually be working on your project, not just the firm.

Before you make a commitment, insist on meeting and evaluating the senior consultant who will lead the team for your project. How long has that person been a consultant and with the firm? What is that individual's project experience? Will that person be on site at appropriate times or just direct from afar? What is that individual's character and competence? Character, capabilities, and competence may be corporate or reflected consistently in the firm's staff members. You want both.

Furthermore, before you make a commitment, you may want to meet other consulting team members and observe the interaction between them and especially between the project manager and more junior personnel. How well do team members interact? If junior people are worshipfully deferential to their boss, or pretend to be, and rarely contribute to the conversation, that tells you one thing. If the boss encourages them to speak up, a manifestation of mentoring, that tells you something else. If the relationships appear stiff rather than comfortable it may suggest that this team has not worked well together before. Ask the junior people what their role will be. Do they know? Does the boss interrupt their response? That may suggest lack of internal communication.

As you consider these issues remember that behavior is influenced by national culture as well as by the internal culture of a consulting organization.

Capabilities

Capabilities are defined by an organization's history of work, typically expressed in a brochure listing completed projects. However, individuals who undertook those projects may no longer be with the organization. Your consulting team consists of individuals who have remained with the company or who were hired after such projects were undertaken. Each individual's working experience is typically expressed in a curriculum vitae which often overstates the individual's accomplishments, just as a corporate brochure or Web site may overstate the accomplishments of an organization.

Are references useful? Perhaps. Asking the prospective consultant for references will obviously get you a very selective list of pleased customers and friends. A better index may be the number of repeat clients, those who have returned to the same firm repeatedly with new projects. Do not hesitate to ask for a list of repeat clients and contacts at these firms.

Competence

There are two parties to a contract and for a project to be successful, both must be competent.

Evaluating and selecting hospital consultants cannot be done well unless you, the client, really understand what you wish to achieve. You must be certain about what you need and you must express your requirements clearly. Sometimes, however, a client will issue a relatively rigid request for proposal (RFP) that specifies direction and tasks in great detail. This may prevent the consultant from offering alternative approaches that deserve your consideration and that may provide better solutions. A tightly written RFP should always contain a clause that encourages the tenderer to present alternative methods and budgets to achieve the same objectives.

The paradox is that when an RFP for highly specialized consulting services is written, it is usually generated by an organization that seeks highly specialized assistance because it lacks the internal capability to do the job itself. It is therefore wise to consult several specialized consultants or other appropriate experts informally before issuing an RFP to learn how they would meet the challenge. If this approach is inappropriate in your environment, consider other alternatives that optimize the RFP. Allow flexibility and ask for alternative approaches.

It is far easier for good consultants to work with knowledgeable clients, and it produces better results faster. If, however, you are hiring a consultant precisely because you lack knowledge of an area, how you relate to the consultant becomes especially important to avoid being exploited. You may wish to require that the consultant explain step-by-step processes and results in real time. It is also important that you appreciate the complexity of health care generally and health care facilities specifically, the value and cost of effective planning, and the strengths and weaknesses of consulting organizations.

How do you determine those strength and weaknesses? What is the depth of the organization's intellectual resources and will they actually be brought to bear on your project? How can you select a consultant that matches the challenge of your project from a technical viewpoint and is also compatible with your national and local environment and organizational culture? Once the choice is made, how can you best work with a consultant to achieve your objectives? What works well and what does not work?

Consultants are hired for several different but not mutually exclusive reasons. Most of the time they are needed for their specialized technical expertise. Sometimes they are needed because personalities in your own organization are in conflict and you want a more objective outsider. Sometimes a consultant is hired simply because your organization lacks the manpower to take on additional tasks. In this case it is important to realize that consultants must also be managed to optimize their focus, productivity, and costs.

Being an Effective Client

To maintain the direction and momentum of a successful project you obviously need that effective consultant. But you also need to be an effective client. How can you be an effective client?

First of all, to maintain your credibility, keep your commitments, both verbal and written, related to meeting dates and times, work review and approval cycles, and payments to the consultant. If you are in a corporate setting in which you lack personal control over these and other issues, make that clear to the consultant in advance. Contractual commitments for payments are sometimes ignored by clients and consultants become disenchanted.

Clients, sometimes slowed by their own internal bureaucracies, often press consultants to begin work before the contractually defined mobilization fees have been paid, arguing that the project is late. Many consultants find that when they do so—in a spirit of cooperation and professional loyalty to a project—their thoughtfulness is punished with further payment delays. They are then "on the hook" and think they cannot stop work.

Consultants usually plan their travel and work schedules to maximize their productivity. They often project their costs based on their expectations about meeting dates and times or when your data or drawings will be given to them or how long it takes to get approvals. In one project a key meeting with senior decision makers in the client's organization was cancelled four times over a two-month period—well beyond the consultant's contractual deadline to complete tasks, but the consultant was still blamed for the delay.

If approvals for completed work or payments must be authorized via a bureaucratic chain of departments and individuals, be sure the consultants understand that approval or payment process and its documentation demands before they commit to a contract, mobilization and progress fees, and schedule. Don't surprise your consultant! In a recent project the consultant followed the instruction of one department in documenting travel expenses for reimbursement, only to be told after months of nonpayment that a different expense reimbursement form was needed.

Do not demand unnecessary or excessive paperwork from your consultants. It wastes their time and your money. If expense reimbursement is contractually on a per diem basis, do not require receipts for hotels, taxis, meals, and incidentals. The purpose of a per diem is to avoid such paperwork and still limit expenses. The reimbursement section of a consultant's contract should specify that the hotel and/or per diem rates for the city in question conform to selected standards (for example, the U.S. Department of State per diem rates).

Consultants can often mobilize and produce results faster than a typical government or private bureaucracy can or will pay for their services. Faced with lagging payments, the consultant, perhaps under pressure from his own chief financial officer, may be told to stop work or may threaten to quit the project. You, the client, perceive this as lack of loyalty to the project and relationship as well as to you personally. The consultant perceives your organization's failure to pay on time as dishonesty, and the relationship is thus poisoned.

Timing becomes an issue. A consultant submits an invited proposal under time pressure ("We have to have it next week!"). Three months go by and the consultant is not contacted with a response. This does not help maintain the overall efficiency of everyone involved.

Finally, remember that consultants are selling their time. Respect that and pay them on time. Trust and loyalty, the foundation of an effective working relationship, must work in both directions.

Appendix G

Typical Provider Payment Mechanisms

Payment mechanism	Unit of service	Determination of payment	Main incentives reported
Fee for service	Per single act or visit	Retrospective	Incentive to increase units of service
Case-based payment, where a fixed sum is paid according to a fee schedule, for example, based on DRGs (diagnosis-related groups); the amount does not necessarily correspond to the actual cost of services or length of stay	Per case or episode	Prospective	Incentive to reduce services per case but increase number of cases (if per-case rate is above marginal costs); incentive to improve efficiency
Per diem	Per day	Prospective	Incentive to reduce services per stay but increase length of stay (if per diem rate is above marginal costs)
Contracting	For a selected group of (or all) services in a given period	Prospective	Varies

Sources: World Health Organization, *Evaluation of Recent Changes in the Financing of Health Services: Report of a WHO Study Group*, WHO Technical Report Series No. 829 (Geneva: World Health Organization, 1993); Daniel Maceira, *Provider Payment Mechanisms in Health Care: Incentives, Outcomes and Organizational Impact in Developing Countries*, Major Applied Research 2, Working Paper 2 (Bethesda, MD: Partnerships for Health Reform Project, Abt Associates, 1998).

Note: When the amount of payment is agreed prior to treatment, the determination of payment is prospective. In these cases the provider faces higher financial risk. When the amount of payment is agreed during or after treatment, the determination is retrospective; this tends to be cost-enhancing.

Appendix H
Different Forms of Business Ownership

Each country has its own laws regulating how businesses may organize their operations, including forms of ownership. This appendix presents brief descriptions of the most common forms of ownership, but it should be kept in mind that there are many different ways to structure the ownership of your hospital in addition to those discussed here. You will have to obtain sufficient information about the laws and regulations in all relevant legal jurisdictions and consult with accounting, tax, and legal advisers before deciding on the ownership form of the hospital. In addition, maintaining well-documented corporate governance records, as well as tax and accounting records, will be critically important.

Sole Proprietorship

A sole proprietorship is a one-person business. Under this structure, you would generally be required to register the facility (as opposed to the owner of the facility) as an operating entity for the purpose of obtaining a business license for a health care facility. The facility itself would hold the license since the owner of the business and the business itself will be one and the same for legal, tax, and other purposes. Because the facility does not have its own legal status, the owner must enter into various contracts, such as employment contracts for staff and workers, in his or her own name. The owner must also report the net income/losses from the facility as his or her own personal income/losses and have them treated as such for tax purposes. Under a sole proprietorship, the owner of the business is personally liable for any business-related financial and other obligations such as debt, contractual obligations and liabilities, and court judgments.

General Partnership

A partnership is a business owned by two or more people who commit to the partnership and its stated objectives and share the benefits and costs of the business. A facility owned by a partnership will be registered in the name of the partnership, which could be the founding members' names or a different name. Each general partner has a legal right to enter into contracts in the partnership's name and bind the partnership to the contracts. However, each partner is personally liable for any claims that might arise against the partnership or any debt the partnership might incur. As in a sole proprietorship, the partnership's owners pay personal income taxes on their respective shares of the business income.

The scope and nature of the partners' responsibilities, both individually and jointly, are governed by a partnership agreement that is signed by all members of the partnership. This agreement is then notarized and registered as a public record. Because of the importance of the partnership agreement, you must ensure that it covers all of the important matters and that each partner has fully understood his or her responsibilities and rights under the agreement before signing it. It should be prepared by your legal counsel at an early stage in project development. Among other matters, it should include provisions for bringing in new partners who may join the partnership at a later stage, as well as releasing those who wish to leave it.

Limited Partnership

A limited partnership is a partnership where the "general partner" is designated as such by agreement. The agreement will detail the functions of the general partner and all limited partners. Generally, a general partner handles the limited partnership's day-to-day operations and is personally liable for its business debt. Limited partners have minimal control over daily business decisions or operations and are not personally liable for business debts or claims. This form of ownership and management structure is most often used for management of investment funds, such as private equity funds. Limited partnerships tend to be costly and are complicated to set up and manage.

Corporation or Limited Liability Company

A corporation is owned by its shareholders. A properly registered corporation is a legal entity, which is governed by the articles of association and bylaws of the corporation adopted by the shareholders. The bylaws dictate how the corporation will operate, for example, who can do what on the corporation's behalf.

This would cover actions such as entering into contractual arrangements, raising financing, hiring people, procuring materials and equipment, and so on. Bylaws should be prepared by your legal counsel to ensure compliance with applicable laws. Shareholders elect the corporation's board of directors but otherwise do not actively manage the corporation. The board of directors usually makes major corporate decisions, while the corporation's officers, who are appointed by the board of directors, conduct the day-to-day management of the business.

Most large businesses operate as corporations, so it is the most familiar form of ownership. The principal appeal of a corporation is that if the corporation gets into financial troubles, the shareholders are liable only to the extent of the capital they have contributed or committed to the corporation, but if the corporation becomes financially successful, the shareholders are entitled to the profits and other values that the business may generate to the extent of each shareholder's ownership percentage. If a corporation has borrowed funds from individuals or institutions and cannot pay them back, the shareholders are not legally liable for the debt unless they themselves have provided guarantees (which could be in various forms) to the lenders or creditors. A single person can be a corporation's owner and sole director and may serve as any officer required by law. A corporation survives the death of a shareholder or other changes in ownership. The main benefit of a corporation is the limit to the owners' personal liability for business liabilities, debts, and court judgments against the business.

Limited liability companies (LLCs) are registered entities that also provide limited liability benefits to their members (owners) but are governed by an operating agreement rather than a set of bylaws. Generally, LLCs have more flexibility in how they are managed. Your legal counsel should draft the operating agreement to ensure all relevant management needs are addressed so that the business will run smoothly. When it comes to taxes, LLCs are often more like partnerships. Generally, the owners of an LLC report their share of business income and/or losses on their personal tax returns and pay taxes on it.

Nonprofit Organization

A nonprofit organization is a legal entity formed to carry out certain activities, including provision of goods and services, on a not-for-profit basis in accordance with the requirements of the relevant jurisdiction's laws and regulations for nonprofit organizations. Usually nonprofit organizations provide services for educational, charitable, religious, or scientific purposes. They typically raise funds by receiving public and private grant monies and donations from individuals and companies. Nonprofit organizations are generally exempt from paying various taxes.

In some countries, private schools and hospitals are required by law to register and operate as nonprofit organizations regardless of market conditions and the types of companies or organizations that operate such institutions. In such a regulatory environment, privately operated schools and hospitals that receive few or no government funds or private grants are still required to register as nonprofits even though they may have to rely on funds generated from their own operations. In many cases, private schools or hospitals may be allowed to take out bank loans, which can be repaid. However, they are prohibited from paying dividends or sharing excess earnings in any other way. If your hospital has to be registered as a nonprofit organization, you will likely experience lack of interest from equity investors. However, each country has its own rules and regulations concerning nonprofit organizations, so you will need to understand them thoroughly before deciding whether to structure the ownership of the facility as nonprofit.

Sole proprietorships and partnerships are generally considered more suitable for small facilities because one or a few persons can take full control of the daily operations. They also tend to be preferable for operations that have a simple business scope, employ few people, do not require much in the way of borrowing, and present limited possibilities for lawsuits.

Appendix I

Sample Project Cost Estimation Summary

Land (m²)	
Building (usable space, m²)	
Beds	

Item	Cost	% of total costs
Land		
Construction (including soft costs and contingency)		
Medical equipment		
Nonmedical equipment, furniture, and fixtures		
MIS/HIS (IT) system		
Project development		
Preopening		
Financing		
Working capital		
TOTAL		100

Item	Unit cost			
	Your hospital	Comparator #1	Comparator #2	Comparator #3
Land (cost/m^2)				
Construction (cost/m^2 land)				
Construction (cost/m^2 built space)				
Construction (cost/bed)				
Nonmedical equipment, furniture, and fixtures (cost/m^2 space)				
Nonmedical equipment, furniture, and fixtures (cost/bed)				
Total project (cost/m^2 land)				
Total project (cost/bed)				
Working capital				

Appendix J

Summary of Project Costs and Financing Plan for a Greenfield Hospital Project

	Project cost			
		Amount in currency needed	*Local currency*	
Item	*Currency*		*Amount*	*%*
Land				
Construction hard costs				
Construction soft costs				
Medical equipment				
Nonmedical equipment				
Furniture, fixtures, and supplies				
IT systems (hardware and software)				
Project development costs				
Preopening costs				
Permanent working capital				
Financing costs				
Contingency				
Total project cost				100

Financing plan				
		Amount in currency needed	Local currency	
Item	Currency		Amount	%
Equity and grants				
Equity, source #1				
Equity, source #2				
Debt financing				
Long-term debt, source #1				
Long-term debt, source #2				
Quasi-equity, source #1				
Total financing				100

Appendix K
Sample Format for a Financial Projection Model

A financial projection model can be structured in many different ways, depending on the project's characteristics and the preferences of the person who will build the model. The following provides selected sections of a projection model. In addition to the formats presented below, additional sections covering financing, capital expenditure, depreciation schedule, return on investment analysis, and ratio analysis will be needed to build a comprehensive financial projection model.

Abbreviations

A&E	accident and emergency
ALOS	average length of stay
CATH LAB	catheterization laboratory
FTE	full-time equivalent
IT	information technology
MIS/HIS	management information system/hospital information system
MRI	magnetic resonance imaging
OT	operating theater

Sample Financial Projections: Market Parameters and Capacity Assumptions

Market parameters	Year 1 (monthly)	Year 2 (monthly)	Year 3	Year 4	Year 5	~Year 10
Population in primary target market (define the area)						
Growth rate						
Population in broader target market (define the area)						
Growth rate						
% of [ ] patients from primary target market						
% of [ ] patients from primary target market						
% of [ ] patients from broader target market						
% of [ ] patients from broader target market						
Primary target market size						
Project's target market size						
Hospitalization market (surgeries, deliveries, medical cases)						
Hospitalization rate per year						
Market pool for project's inpatient services						
% of patients hospitalized for surgery						
% of patients hospitalized for delivery						
% of patients hospitalized for medical service						
Project's market pool for surgeries						
Project's market pool for deliveries						
Project's market pool for medical cases						
Medical visits market						
Medical visits per person per year						
Project's market pool for medical visits						
Endoscopy market						
Endoscopy rate as % of medical visits						
Project's market pool for endoscopy						

Capacity assumptions	Year 1 (monthly)	Year 2 (monthly)	Year 3	Year 4	Year 5	~Year 10
Total number of beds						
# of inpatient beds, of which:						
– # of beds for surgeries						
– # of beds for deliveries						
– # of beds for medical cases						
# of intensive care unit beds						
# of beds for ambulatory surgeries						
# of beds for chemotherapy						
# of operating theaters						
# of delivery wards						
# of imagery equipment (radiology)						

Sample Financial Projections: Key Assumptions for Operation

	Year 1 (monthly)	Year 2 (monthly)	Year 3	Year 4	Year 5
Maximum capacity rate					
Surgeries					
Market share achievable					
Potential market					
Maximum # of admission days for surgeries	365 days				
Maximum # of inpatients	ALOS (days)				
Maximum # of ambulatory surgeries	# per bed per year				
Maximum capacity of operating theaters	# per OT per year				
	of total # surgery				
# of ambulatory surgeries	of total # surgery				
# of surgeries					
Growth rate					
Market share—surgeries					
Inpatient surgery days					
Inpatient beds' utilization rate (%)					
Outpatient beds' utilization rate (%)					
OT utilization rate (%)					
Deliveries					
Market share achievable					
Potential market					
Maximum # of beds available for deliveries per year					
Maximum # of deliveries in wards per year	deliveries per ward per year				
# of deliveries					
Growth rate					
Market share—deliveries					
# of deliveries days	ALOS (days)				
Beds' capacity utilization (%)					
Ward capacity utilization (%)					
Medical cases					
Market share achievable					
Potential market					
Maximum # of medical days	365 days				
Maximum # of medical cases					
# of medical cases					
Growth rate					
Market share—medical cases					
# of medical days	ALOS (days)				
Beds' capacity utilization (%)					
Day hospital—other					
Endoscopy					
Potential market	% of potential medical visits				
Maximum # of patients in endoscopy	per year				
# of patients in endoscopy					
Market share					
Capacity utilization (%)					
Lithotripsy					
Potential market					
Maximum # of patients in lithotripsy					
# of patients in lithotripsy					
Capacity utilization (%)					

Sample Financial Projections: Key Assumptions for Operation (continued)

		Year 1 (monthly)	Year 2 (monthly)	Year 3	Year 4	Year 5
Medical visits						
Market share achievable						
Potential market						
Maximum # of medical visits	per year					
# of medical visits						
Growth rate						
Market share						
Capacity utilization (%)						
Other						
Chemotherapy and radiotherapy						
Potential treatment market	# of visits per patient					
Maximum # of chemotherapy/radiotherapy treatments						
# of chemotherapy/radiotherapy treatments						
Capacity utilization (%)						
X-ray and scanner						
Paying x-ray and scanner patients	% of medical visits					
Packages including x-ray and scanner	% of medical visits					
Maximum # of x-ray and scanner images	# of images per machine per day					
Capacity utilization (%)						

Sample Financial Projections: Revenue Assumptions

	Year 1 (monthly)	Year 2 (monthly)	Year 3	Year 4	Year 5
Price increase					
Multiplier for sensitivity analysis: 1					
Sensitvity: % discount for late start of operations					
* % price discounts and pro-bono for social service*					

Inpatients
# of inpatients
Average length of stay

Inpatient surgeries
# of surgeries
Price for surgeries
Revenue from surgery

Deliveries
# of deliveries   charge per delivery
Revenue from maternity

Medical cases
# of medical cases   charge per case
Revenue from medical cases

Revenues from inpatients

Day hospital
# of patients in day hospital

Ambulatory surgery
# of ambulatory surgeries
Revenue from ambulatory surgery $ per surgery

Endoscopy
# of patients in endoscopy
Revenue from endoscopy $ per procedure

Lithotripsy
# of patients in lithotripsy
Revenue from lithotripsy $ per procedure

Revenues from day hospital

Outpatients
# of outpatients including health card patients
# of outpatients excluding health card patients

Medical visits and A&E
# of patients in medical visits and A&E
# of patients in medical visits and A&E excluding health card
Revenue from medical visits $ per visit

Chemotherapy and radiotherapy
# of chemotherapy/radiotherapy treatments
Revenue from chemotherapy/radiotherapy $ per visit

Sample Financial Projections: Revenue Assumptions (continued)

		Year 1 (monthly)	Year 2 (monthly)	Year 3	Year 4	Year 5
Revenues from outpatients						
Radiology and laboratory						
X-ray and scanner						
# of x-ray and scanner tests						
Revenue from x-ray and scanner	$ per test					
MRI						
# of MRI examinations						
Revenue from MRI	$ per procedure					
Catheterization laboratory (CATH LAB)						
# of CATH LAB procedures						
Revenue from CATH LAB	$ per procedure					
Laboratory						
# of patients getting laboratory tests	% of medical visits					
Revenue from laboratory	$ per patient					
Revenues from radiology and laboratory						
Pharmacy						
Revenue from pharmacy	% of total revenue					
Other						
Other service/product line						
# of units	% of outpatients					
Revenue from other service/product	$ per unit					
Extra charges for suites						
# of patients in suites	% of inpatients					
# of patient days in suites						
Revenue from suite charges	$ per suite day					
Other sources						
Revenue from other sources	basis to be determined					
Other revenues						

Sample Financial Projections: Summary of Revenues

	Year 1 (monthly)		Year 2 (monthly)		Year 3		Year 4		Year 5	
	Amount	%	Amount	%	Amount	%	Amount	%	Amount	%
Revenues from inpatients										
Inpatient surgery										
Maternity										
Medical cases										
Revenues from day hospital										
Ambulatory surgery										
Endoscopy										
Lithotripsy										
Revenues from outpatients										
Medical visits										
Oncology										
Revenues from radiology										
Revenues from laboratory										
Revenues from pharmacy										
Other revenues										
Total revenues										

Sample Financial Projections: Estimation of Costs

			Year 1 (monthly)	Year 2 (monthly)	Year 3	Year 4	Year 5
Cost increase							
Multiplier: 1							
% discount for late start of operations							
Employment costs							
Doctors							
# of local doctors	# normal opening						
# of expatriate doctors (if applicable)	# normal opening						
Total # of doctors	# minimum						
# of medical procedures							
maximum # of procedures per doctor							
Salary plus benefits and taxes per doctor		*Cost increase*					
Local doctors	per month	Y					
Expatriate doctors (if applicable)	$ per month	Y					
Medical and medical support staff							
# of nurses	per bed						
# of FTE staff (other than nurses)	per bed						
# of medical and administration staff including nurses							
Average annual cost (salary, benefits, and taxes) per nurse							
Average annual cost per nonmedical staff							
Corporate support and administrative staff							
# of corporate support staff (accounting, IT support, and others)							
# of marketing and corporate relations staff							
Total # of corporate support and marketing staff							
Average annual cost (salary, benefits, and taxes) per staff							
Executive staff and department heads							
Chief executive officer	per month	Y					
Chief financial officer	per month	Y					
Medical director	per month	Y					
Nursing director	per month	Y					
Other directors	per month						
Other employee-related expenses							
Training	annual cost per staff						
Travel for executive staff	# of travels per year						
Total travel cost	cost per trip	Y					
Total employment costs							

Sample Financial Projections: Estimation of Costs (continued)

			Year 1 (monthly)	Year 2 (monthly)	Year 3	Year 4	Year 5
Medical, pharmaceutical, and nonmedical supplies							
Medical and pharmaceutical supplies							
Oxygen and medical gases	$ maximum # of OT	N					
Drugs and disposables	$ per surgery	Y					
	$ per maternity	Y					
	$ per medical case	Y					
	$ per medical visit	Y					
	$ per chemotherapy	Y					
	$ per radiology	Y					
	% of pharmacy revenue						
Blood	$ per surgery	Y					
Laboratory tests	$ per health card patient						
Protheses and implants	$ per prosthesis	Y					
	# of surgeries						
Other supplies							
Food supplies	$ per inpatient day	N					
Linen and ward supplies	$ per bed per year	N					
Supplies for annex activities	% of revenue other sources	Y					
Other supplies	$	N					
Outsourcing fees (if applicable, by type)							
Total medical, pharmaceutical, and nonmedical supplies							
General and administrative costs							
Management fees—base (if applicable)							
Management fees—incentive (if applicable)							
Consultant fees		Y					
Land lease							
Utilities		N					
Insurance		Y					
Telecommunications charges		Y					
Maintenance costs - building		N					
- housing complex		Y					
- as % of total building value							
Equipment maintenance cost amount		N					
Equipment maintenance as % of total equipment cost							
MIS/HIS maintenance and upgrades							
Office supplies							
Training expenses							
Travel expenses							
Legal counsel's fees		N					
Auditors' fees		N					
Other service fees		N					
Social fund contribution							
Bad debts	% of revenues or some other basis						
Total sales, general, and administrative expenses							

Sample Financial Projections: Income Statements

	Year 1 (monthly)	Year 2 (monthly)	Year 3	Year 4	Year 5	~ Year 10
Revenues						
Inpatients						
Day hospital						
Outpatients						
Diagnostic services						
Pharmacy						
Other revneues						
Total revenues						
Operating supplies						
Medical supplies						
Pharmaceutical supplies						
Nonmedical supplies						
Office and other supplies						
Cost of operating supplies						
Total operating supplies						
Operating expenses						
Staff costs						
Salaries						
Benefits (medical insurance, pension, taxes, and so forth)						
Subtotal: staff costs						
Staff training expenses						
Staff travelling expenses						
Medical equipment maintenance						
IT systems maintenance and upgrades						
Building and fixtures' maintenance						
Management service fees (if applicable)						
Outsourcing fees (if applicable)						
Rental charges (if applicable)						
Marketing and corporate development						
Utilities						
Insurance						
Telecommunications						
Professional fees						
Social fund contribution (if applicable)						
Bad debts						
Miscellaneous						
Total operating expenses						
Earnings before interest, taxes, depreciation, and amortization						
Cash operating margin before financial charges and taxes (%)						
Depreciation and amortization						
Earnings before interest and taxes						
Financial charges						
Leasing charges (if applicable)						
Net income before tax and extraordinary items						
Foreign exchange gains/losses (if applicable)						
Extraordinary items						
Corporate income tax						
Net income						
Net cash margin (%)						

Sample Financial Projections: Balance Sheet

	Year 1 (monthly)	Year 2 (monthly)	Year 3	Year 4	Year 5	~ Year 10
Assets						
Current assets						
Cash in bank and in hand						
Cash in bank—pension fund or other special purpose (with restricted withdrawal conditions)						
Accounts receivable						
Inventories						
Prepaid expenses						
Deposits						
Total current assets						
Fixed assets						
Land						
Buildings (including soft costs)						
Infrastructure						
Fixtures and furniture						
Medical equipment						
IT system						
(Deduct: accumulated depreciation and amortization)						
Net fixed assets						
Other long-term assets						
Total assets						
Liabilities and shareholders' equity						
Current liabilities						
Accounts payables						
Current portion of long-term debt						
Taxes payable						
Other payables						
Total current liabilities						
Long-term liabilities						
Long-term debt						
Long-term quasi-equity						
Capitalized leasing charges (if applicable)						
Pension fund liability (if applicable)						
Total long-term liabilities						
Total liabilities						
Shareholders' equity						
Paid-in capital						
Capital reserves (including grants)						
Accumulated retained earnings (losses)						
Current period's profit/loss						
Total shareholders' equity						
Total liabilities and shareholders' equity						

Sample Financial Projections: Cash Flow Statement

	Year 1 (monthly)	Year 2 (monthly)	Year 3	Year 4	Year 5	~ Year 10
Cash flow from operations						
Net income						
Plus (minus):						
Financial charges						
Noncash extraordinary items						
Depreciation and amortization						
Provision for bad debts						
Foreign currency translation losses (gains)						
Other noncash items						
Cash flow from operations						
Net changes in working capital						
Cash flow from operations after working capital changes						
Cash flow from investment activities						
Capital expenditure						
Sale (disposal) of hard assets						
Other						
Cash flow from investment activities						
Free cash flow available for debt service and dividends						
Cash flow from financing activities						
Debt financing and debt service:						
Debt and quasi-equity financing received						
Debt and quasi-equity financing repaid						
Adjustments to debt						
Interest and other financial charges paid						
Revenues/income-sharing charges paid (if applicable)						
Net cash flow from debt financing activities						
Equity-related financing:						
Capital subscription/increases						
Grants						
Dividends paid						
Redemption of preferred shares (if applicable)						
Other						
Net cash flow from equity financing activities						
Cash flow from financing activities						
Net cash flow during the period						
Cash balance—beginning						
Cash balance—ending						
Less: restricted cash (for example, for pension)						
Cash balance—ending and available for use						

Appendix L

Sample Outline for a Business Plan

I. Executive Summary

A. Project concept, mission, and objectives
  1. Explain the project's concept, mission (if a mission statement has been prepared), and main objectives.

B. Project summary
  1. Summarize the project, including its background, sponsors, long-term (or master) plan and its phasing, physical features, target markets, particular strengths, total project cost, financial plan, timing of construction and opening, projected operational and financial performance, and other highlights.

C. Project owners (sponsors) and project management team
  1. List the project owners and the background of each individual or legal entity. Describe the ownership structure of the project company and note the amount of funds the owners will invest in the company.
  2. Explain who will manage the project's planning and construction and who will manage the hospital after it begins operation.

D. Project status and next steps
  1. Summarize progress made to date concerning the prefeasibility study, market research, any permits received or applied for, steps toward obtaining land, amount of funds raised and spent, and so on.

II. Political, Economic, and Regulatory Environment (National and Regional)

A. Basic characteristics
   1. For the country and region, describe population size and composition by age and gender, geographic characteristics, natural resources, major industries, and other relevant information.

B. Political environment
   1. Explain the country's political system, political trends and government stability, and administration of the health care sector at the national and regional levels.

C. Economic and business environment
   1. Describe income levels, employment levels, and major economic activities; the structure of the banking sector and nonbank financial services sector (such as leasing industry); the insurance industry; government policies and priorities regarding economic growth; and economic trends.

D. Legal and regulatory environment
   1. Explain existing laws and regulations affecting the health care sector, businesses, financing, and foreign investment. These may include requirements and procedures relating to licensing of hospitals and medical personnel, health and safety, medical accidents and malpractice, administration of food and drugs, environmental matters, labor management, approval of foreign investment, ownership of health care facilities, various taxes applicable to the project, any incentives, and others.

E. Changes expected in the next 3–5 years

III. Health Status and the Health Care Industry (National and Regional)

A. Overview of health status and demand for health care
   1. Provide an overview, at the national level, of the population's health status (compare to relevant countries, if useful), epidemiology, major diseases and medical needs, major gaps in the provision of health care services (that is, unmet demands), government budget for health care by category, estimated average annual spending for health care by

households, and how people obtain health care. Assess major issues, recent trends, and changes expected.

2. Provide the same overview for the region and/or areas that are target markets of the project. Provide quantified assessments to the extent possible.

B. Provision of health care services
   1. Provide a table summarizing total number of health care facilities, nationally and regionally, by type of facility (hospitals, clinics, specialty facilities, and so on) and by type of ownership and management (public, private for-profit, private not-for-profit).
   2. Describe the structure and particular characteristics of the health care industry, patient referral system, medical personnel education and training system, and health insurance system, and their impact on health care provision. Assess major issues, recent trends, and changes expected.

C. Public hospitals
   1. Explain services provided, average conditions of facilities, major characteristics, number of patients cared for annually, prices charged, any issues relating to collection of service charges, budgets received, staffing issues, financial conditions, and special services offered to increase revenues. Assess key issues, recent trends (including any public-private partnerships), government plans for change in the next 3–5 years, and likelihood that planned changes will be implemented.

D. Private health care facilities
   1. Provide the same assessment described above for any private hospitals in the country or region.

E. Health care insurance
   1. Describe the existing health insurance programs, how they work, pricing, payment terms, insurance coverage, level of participation, any particular issues, and changes anticipated.

F. Changes expected in the next 3–5 years

IV. The Project: Markets, Operation, and Management

A. Target markets
   1. Define and quantify the target markets by geographic boundaries and any specific characteristics.

2. Describe demographics, epidemiology, and medical needs in the target markets.
3. In a table, list the hospitals that exist or are planned in your target markets. Identify those that would likely be competitors to your hospital, including ones that are located outside your target markets but could offer competition because of, for example, their specialty. Discuss the history, ownership, facilities, management, occupancy rates, operating and financial performance, pricing policies and practices, and competitive strengths and weaknesses of each competitor institution.
4. Explain your hospital's competitive strengths in view of its competition.
5. Articulate recent tends in the demand and supply situation in your target markets and discuss changes anticipated in the next 3–5 years.

B. Project stakeholders
1. Elaborate on the information in part I, section C, regarding the project's community, public parties, private sector partners if any, and other relevant information.

C. Medical operations
1. Describe services to be offered during each phase of the project.
2. Describe the functional programs for the first phase and those for the second phase. Note whether the second phase is to occur soon after the first phase for each function, and explain how the functions have been selected. The functions could include the following: anesthesiology and operating suite; accident and emergency; intensive care unit; inpatient department; outpatient department; imaging department; surgical specialties; oncology; interventional cardiology; maternity; pharmacy; laboratory; blood bank; laundry, sterilization, and kitchen; or other support functions.

D. Operating plan
1. Explain how the hospital will gain access to patients.
2. Describe the target patient mix and volume. Provide projections (monthly for the first two years of operation, annually thereafter) for each service and operating unit.
3. Explain the target average length of stay, how it is projected to change over time, and related aspects.
4. Explain treatment protocols, operating policies and procedures, and languages to be used.
5. Outline prices planned for each procedure or service (or package of procedures/services). Discuss how prices have been determined, how prices compare to those charged by potential competitors (both within

the country and abroad, if applicable), and any issues related to pricing.

6. Discuss average revenues targeted per patient and per procedure (or package of procedures/services, if applicable) and how they are expected to change over time.

7. Discuss plans for social services for low-income and/or nonpaying patients.

E. Organization and management

1. Explain the operating company and the ownership structure of the hospital and the operating company.

2. Present diagrams for the organizational structure of the project planning and management team and of the hospital management (for operation). Elaborate on the plans for management summarized in part I, section C.

F. Staffing and training

1. Explain the composition of medical staff, where will they come from, and the timing of recruitment.

2. Estimate average salary, benefits, and taxes per medical staff member (separately for doctors and nurses, and for local staff and expatriates, if applicable).

3. Present the same information for nonmedical staff.

4. Explain certification and licensing requirements.

5. Discuss staff training plans and costs.

G. Marketing

1. Articulate the marketing strategy, marketing plans, programs, activities, staffing, cost estimates, and other relevant information, for each stage of the project's planning, construction, and operation.

V. The Project: Facility and Construction

A. Site

1. Explain the location and ownership of the site.

2. Describe its physical setting, natural environment (and any potential for natural disasters), geotechnical conditions, and proximity to major industrial or other facilities. Describe access to utilities and access to the site (roads and bridges, if any, and availability of public transportation to the site).

3. Present a map.

B. Facility design
   1. Present the schematic design and explain its status (draft or final).
   2. Explain key aspects of the design, including the architect, the design process, and what more needs to be done.

C. Construction plans
   1. Present construction plans in detail, including phases, critical milestones, timetable, estimated hard and soft costs, material sourcing, use of professional services, construction management team, likely contractors and their backgrounds, unresolved issues, and key risks.

D. Construction management team
   1. Describe the construction planning and management team.

E. Medical equipment
   1. List medical equipment planned and explain the types of equipment planned, likely suppliers, medical equipment planner, status of discussions/negotiations, likelihood of changes, scope of services by suppliers, plans for equipment installation and commissioning and maintenance, as well as supplies needed to operate the equipment, who will supply them, and associated costs.

F. Information technology (IT) and telecommunications systems
   1. Explain what kind of IT and telecom systems will be installed, the technology, the supplier, costs, and any potential issues.

G. Management information system for a hospital information system (MIS/HIS)
   1. Explain the plans for MIS/HIS system procurement, implementation, and maintenance, including who will supply the system, what kind of package will be procured, cost, supplier's responsibilities, supplier's background and track record, installation timetable, status of negotiations, and who will handle this matter among the members of the project management team.

H. Construction timetable and start-up plans
   1. Explain construction timetable (present more than one timetable, if necessary, to account for contingent events). Note milestones, including installation of IT and telecom systems, medical equipment, kitchen and other facilities, and other important steps.
   2. Explain plans for hospital commissioning, dry runs, and starting of phase I services.

I. Facility management plans
   1. Explain the scope of maintenance needs for the buildings, medical and other equipment, IT systems, and MIS/HIS system after the hospital's opening. Discuss arrangements to be made to address needs and costs.

J. Environmental and safety issues
   1. Explain all issues related to environmental protection (especially medical waste treatment) and worker safety. Discuss how each issue will be managed and the costs associated with management.

VI. The Project: Financial Aspects

A. Project cost
   1. Present a table detailing each component of the project cost by category (hard and soft costs, fees by type, preopening expenses, permanent working capital). Discuss contingencies and the timing of cash payments.

B. Financial plan
   1. Explain the financial plan, noting each category of financing being sought and different capitalization scenarios, if applicable. Note how much funding has been raised so far and on what terms and conditions, and how much is expected to be raised from whom, on what terms and conditions, and in what time frame. Note how much has been spent and for what purposes. Discuss cash flow estimates and potential changes and issues.

C. Operational and financial projections
   1. Present a summary of financial projections.
   2. Explain details of assumptions used to project the levels of operation of each department or service unit, as well as details of projected revenues and expenses.
   3. Present projected financial statements, that is, income statement, cash flow statement, and balance sheet, in detail, with monthly projections for the first two years of operations and quarterly projections for years three and four (and annual projections from year five on).
   4. Explain various taxes applicable to the project and the hospital's operation, including income taxes, remittance taxes, interest withholding taxes, business registration tax, value-added taxes, and any others. Explain the loss carry-over regulations in the country.

D. Summary of financial viability and sensitivity scenarios
  1. Present the internal rate of return on total investment.
  2. Present the base case financial projections and various sensitivity scenarios based on revisions to key assumptions, particularly in relation to risks that are identified as beyond the control of the project's sponsors and the hospital's management.
  3. Explain changes in the assumptions used for the sensitivity cases, the implications of each sensitivity scenario, the likelihood of each scenario becoming a reality, and actions that can be prepared to manage the situation in the event it occurs.
  4. Presented selected financial ratios such as the current ratio, asset turnover ratio, debt-to-asset ratio, and debt-to-equity ratio, as well as profitability measures (cash margins at different levels, return on assets, return on equity, and so forth) for base case and sensitivity cases.

VII. The Project: Risk Assessment and Management

A. Country risks
  1. Explain various risks related to the national environment. For each identified risk, note the current situation, likelihood that the risk will materialize, and potential ways that the risk could be prevented, minimized, transferred to other parties, or otherwise dealt with effectively. Identify risks that cannot be avoided or minimized and to which the project (during construction) and the hospital (after opening) will therefore be exposed. Examples of country-related risks include, but are not limited to:
     - Social and/or political instability
     - Approvals and licensing (authorities and procedures)
     - Price controls
     - Issues relating to financing
     - Currency devaluation
     - Foreign exchange control policies and lack of availability of hard currencies
     - Restrictions on the repatriation and remittance of profits
     - Changes in laws and regulations (including rules related to insolvency)
     - Administrative formalities, social customs, and so forth
     - Dispute resolution mechanisms (or lack thereof)

B. Project risks
  1. Explain various project-related risks, giving the same information as described above. Examples of project-related risks include, but are not limited to:
      • Construction delays, cost overruns, and construction quality problems
      • Management problems
      • Language problems
      • Planning problems and start-up delays
      • Staffing problems and labor relations issues
      • Slow revenue generation (slow build-up of operating activities)
      • Operating cost overruns
      • Medical complications, medical and hospital malpractice (related to this is lack of compliance with medical protocols and other operating policies and guidelines)
      • Shortage of power, water, and medical gases and fluids
      • Lack of critical supplies
      • Marketing problems
      • Maintenance issues
      • Environmental and safety risks
      • Thefts in various forms

C. Insurable risks
  1. Provide an overview of insurable risks in terms of the availability of insurance coverage in the country and the types of insurance policies that are available for purchase. Cover the follow areas:
      • Construction-related: all risk insurance, advance loss of profits insurance, cargo insurance, start-up delay insurance
      • Operation-related: all risk insurance, malpractice insurance, business interruption insurance, machinery breakdown insurance, workers compensation insurance, public liability insurance, professional liability insurance, motor vehicle insurance, medical and evacuation insurance

D. Identified but unavoidable and uninsurable risks
  1. List and explain the key risks that are assessed to be relevant to the hospital's construction and operation but that cannot be avoided, insured, or managed in any other way. Assess the likelihood that each such risk will become a reality, the trigger events, and the level of impact that each such risk could have on the hospital's operation and finances.

VIII. The Project: Current Status and Next Steps

A. Current status
1. Explain the status of the project to date, covering all key aspects, including the following:
   - Consultations held with relevant communities and other stakeholders
   - Facility planning completed (assess likelihood that facility design will change)
   - Site acquisition, land ownership registration, and geotechnical analysis completed
   - Construction preparations made
   - Equipment ordered and/or delivered to the project site
   - Approvals secured (for medical operation, investment, and technology importation and installation, and so forth), and licenses and permits received and/or submitted for approval
   - Number of people hired
   - Contracts signed
   - Operating policies and procedures written
   - Registration of legal entities completed (both within the project country and in other countries, if applicable)
   - Amount of funds raised and spent
   - Written commitments obtained from potential investors

B. Next steps
1. Explain next steps planned and needed to move forward with the project. Cover aspects listed above as well as any other matters relevant to the project, with the estimated timing of each step or milestone.

Appendix M
Selected Examples of Financing Sources

Sources of finance	Type of finance	Public sector	Not-for-profit	For-profit
Medical equipment financing firms				
GE Capital Healthcare Financial Services	Loans, leasing		••	••
Philips Medical Systems	Loans, leasing	••	••	••
Siemens	Loans, leasing, equity	••	••	••
Investment funds				
Latin Healthcare Fund	Equity			••
Development Finance Limited, Caribbean	Equity, loans			••
Small Enterprise Assistance Funds (SEAF)	Equity, loans, technical assistance			••
International financial institutions				
African Development Bank	Grants, loans, equity	••	•	•
Asian Development Bank	Grants, loans, equity	••	•	•
European Community	Grants	••	•	
Inter-American Development Bank	Loans	••		•
Inter-American Investment Corporation	Loans, equity		•	••
International Finance Corporation	Loans, equity		•	••
Multilateral Investment Fund	Grants, loans, equity, TA	••	••	••
World Bank	Loans	••		

Sources of finance	Type of finance	Public sector	Not-for-profit	For-profit
Bilateral assistance programs				
Australian Agency for International Development (AusAID)	Grants	••	••	•
Canadian International Development Agency (CIDA)	Grants	••	••	•
UK Department for International Development	Grants	••	••	•
German Agency for Technical Cooperation (GTZ)	Grants	••	••	•
Japan Bank for International Cooperation (JBIC)	Loans, equity	••		••
Japan International Cooperation Agency (JICA)	Grants	••	•	
Kreditanstalt für Wiederaufbau (KfW)	Grants, loans	••	••	••
U.S. Agency for International Devleopment	Grants	••	••	•
U.S. Export-Import Bank	Loans			••
Bilateral investment funds				
American Enterprise Funds	Loans, equity			••
CDC Capital Partners	Loans, equity			••
Overseas Private Investment Corporation (OPIC)	Loans, loan guarantees		•	••
OPIC-supported investment funds	Equity			••
Foundations				
Bill & Melinda Gates Foundation	Grants		••	
David & Lucile Packard Foundation	Grants		••	
Ford Foundation	Grants, loans, equity, loan guarantees	••	••	
Hewlett Foundation	Grants	•	••	
MacArthur Foundation	Grants, loans, equity	•	••	
Mellon Foundation	Grants	•	••	
Rockefeller Foundation	Grants, fellowships		••	

•• = Major recipient of financing; • = Minor recipient of financing

Source: Summa Foundation, *Financing for the Private Health Sector*, Summa Private Sector Tools Series, No. 1 (Washington, DC: Summa Foundation, 2002).

Appendix N
Additional Information on Preferred Shares

Redemption rights can be structured in ways similar to the ways in which repayments of a loan are determined, that is, in a lump sum, a one-time payment, or installments. A redemption right provides an equity investor with a way to exit from the investment. The lump-sum payment for redemption of the shares can be negotiated in different ways, including a sum equal to the amount of the original investment, an amount that includes the original capital plus a certain rate of return, or an amount that is determined according to a certain formula. If the redemption is decided based on a formula, there is no guarantee that the final amount will be greater than the original investment. Instead, there is a possibility that it could be less than the amount of the original investment, which means that the investor shares the risk that the company's future performance could be lower than initially expected. If and when a redemption right is structured as a formula, it is better to state clearly the details of the formula at the time of the agreement, rather than leaving the details to future negotiations.

Two or more of the features described above can be combined to structure an issuance of preferred shares in a wide variety of ways. For example, the shares can be designed as nonredeemable preferred shares with predetermined dividend payments only, or as nonredeemable preferred shares with special dividend payments and higher (than common shares) ranking of recovery upon liquidation and/or financial restructuring. If you agree to redemption rights, then the shares would become redeemable preferred shares with special rights to preferential dividends and/or priority over common shares in case of liquidation of the company.

A conversion right would give the shareholder the right to convert preferred shares, which are often (but not always) nonvoting, into voting common shares. Thus, a preferred share can be designed as, for example, a convertible preferred share with special rights to dividends and/or higher ranking over common shares at the time of liquidation. Note that when the conversion rights are exercised, it would cause an increase in the total number of common shares issued and outstanding and a change in the ownership percentages. By agreeing to give a conversion right to an investor, you would be exposing your ownership rights and those of your partners to potential dilution. Therefore, you will need to consider the possible dilution effect before agreeing to specifics of such arrangements.

The structure of a preferred share that would give an investor the most incentives would be a voting, convertible, redeemable preferred share with rights to mandatory dividend payments. However, such a structure would be more valuable to an investor than a typical loan, considering the difference in the structure of a security package for the loan. Therefore, such a structure would represent a much higher cost to the receiver of the financing. In addition, financing arrangements with complicated structures generally cost substantially more to negotiate and document. You will need to consider the merits of structuring equity financing in different ways and look for ways to keep the structure simple while trying to satisfy the investors' demands to the extent possible.

Appendix O

Programming Individual Departments or Services

When you initiate the general programming for a facility, you will make broad decisions as to the extent of services and the mode of operation. These decisions, which are made for the facility as a whole, form the basis for the detailed planning of every service and service area. The goal is to produce a well-coordinated and efficiently operating facility. The following steps are suggested as an approach to programming individual service areas.

Step 1

Review the functions and decide the general policies and procedures for the operation of the service area. This can be done by determining:

- Types of functions for which provisions will be made in each service area
- Processes by which each function will be carried out
- Which staff member(s) will be responsible for each function
- Types of equipment, furniture, and supplies needed to carry out each function

In some instances, the general policies and procedures for a service area may not differ from those for the facility as a whole. For example, it may have been previously decided that linens will be stored on the carts and delivered to the various service areas and no fixed shelves are needed. Therefore, it may not be necessary to further refine the plan for storing and distributing linen. Instead, the size of the cart needed and the clean area where the linens are to be stored within the service area should be determined.

There are also instances where further determination of policies and procedures is required. For instance, it may have been determined that all preparation of surgical and obstetrical supplies and equipment will be carried out in a central service function. In the planning of the surgery suite, there is a need to formulate policies and procedures for collecting and sending the supplies and equipment to the central service and for storing the supplies and equipment once they have been cleaned. These policies and procedures will set out the amount of space and the type of equipment necessary for this workflow.

Step 2

Determine the rooms or different work areas that are needed. The numbers and types of rooms should be determined through the study of the functions and the policies and procedures which have been formulated in step 1. Functions may be grouped together according to their logical relationship. The following groupings may indicate what functions should be carried out in the same rooms and which functions should be carried out in separate rooms:

- Technique
- Volume of work
- Best work flow
- Personnel responsible for each function
- Types of certain equipment serving more than one function

Step 3

Determine the relationships between departments and services. Decide how the various rooms and areas within the service area should be located in relationship to one another. Logical traffic and workflow would be determining factors in deciding which rooms should be adjacent and which should be located in specific areas. It may not be possible to achieve architecturally ideal relationships so it would be best to indicate the most important items to which the architect should give preference.

Step 4

Determine the design criteria for each room or area. This final step in programming requires a detailed study of work organization within each room. The following steps are suggested as a means of programming the requirements for each room.

- List the functions to be carried out in the room.
- Study activities and determine workstations.
- Determine the activities or subdivisions of work that are necessary to accomplish each function that is to be carried out in the room.
- Decide which of these activities can be handled at the same workstation and which will require separate workstations.
- Determine the equipment for each workstation. The listing of equipment required at each workstation should include: (a) fixed equipment such as work counters, cabinets, sinks, other stationary equipment; (b) mobile equipment that will be kept or used within the room, such as a portable ultrasound machine. It is important that the architect understand the different types of mobile equipment so that he or she makes space for it to be conveniently located in the work area in which it is to be used. If the architect does not have a clear picture, then the equipment could end up blocking the workspace or traffic and interfering with the efficient functioning of the room. Even something as seemingly small as a dirty linen container can present a problem if there is no space to properly locate it.
- Decide on working relationships within the room. Work flow charts can be used to help determine these relationships.
- Determine how the different workstations in the room should be located in relationship to each other. Can they be adjoining or should they have a definite physical separation? Is there any equipment that will serve more than one workstation and therefore should be located between the workstations?
- Decide how the different items of equipment within each workstation should be located in relationship to one another. For instance, should a sink be located at the end of a work counter or in the middle of a work counter?

Step 5

Determine other special requirements for the room. Items that might require special consideration include:

- Special plumbing requirements
- Oxygen outlets
- Vacuum outlets
- Compressed air outlets

- Pressure requirements (for instance, for pressurized rooms)
- Gas outlets
- Waste gas evacuation system
- Special lighting
- Electrical outlets
- Ventilation
- Communications
- Finishes
- Entry and exit requirements
- Special design requirements

It is important to note where special features in equipment are necessary for proper work conditions. For instance, in some areas such as the hospital central service and the laboratory, where personnel do a lot of work in a sitting position, it is important to provide adequate knee space or a footrest. In some areas it may be desirable to design the space so that the staff can alternate between standing and sitting and thus avoid fatigue. Here is a partial list of suggested services to be considered in the functional program:

- *Administrative:* lobby, administrative offices, business and accounting facilities, personnel department, admitting, switchboard, reception
- *Support services:* communications, supplies, stores, laundry, plant engineering and maintenance, housekeeping, materials management, dietary, central services
- *Specialized services:* pharmacy, medication distribution, medical records, social services, spiritual services
- *Nursing and medical services:* utility room, exam rooms, diagnostic and treatment rooms, specialized medical procedure rooms
- *Educational services:* education for patients and their families; in-service staff training and continuing education and staff meetings
- *Miscellaneous services and auxiliary functions:* gift shop, conference rooms, libraries, cafeteria

Here is a list of suggested systems to be considered:

Mechanical, plumbing, and electrical systems

- Chilled water distribution
- Heating/hot water distribution
- Steam distribution
- Air distribution (HVAC)
- Domestic water systems (hot and cold)

- Positive/negative pressure rooms
- Medical gas systems: pumps, compressors, and so forth
- Fire protection systems
- Plumbing systems: fixtures, valves, hardware, and so forth
- Main electrical service and evaluation of existing loads and capacity for future expansions/renovations
- Distribution systems including main switchgear, subpanels, and disconnects
- Emergency service and evaluation of existing loads and capacity for future expansions/renovations
- Fire alarm system
- Call systems
- Elevators
- Security
- Existing code-related deficiencies for the intended use of the facility
- Estimate of remaining useful life and costs to replace/repair equipment

Medical communications systems

- Telephone system (including wireless)
- Hospital information system (HIS)
- Voice and data infrastructure
- Telemedicine, teleradiology, and picture archiving and communicating system (PACs) (network infrastructure)
- Patient monitoring and telemetry (network infrastructure)
- Nurse call/code blue
- Pocket paging
- Staff/patient/visitor equipment location
- Public address
- Theater/auditorium sound
- Intercom
- Radio (two-way and ambulance)
- Dictation and transcription
- Cable/satellite television
- Videoconferencing
- Education and entertainment video distribution
- Audio/video presentation
- Closed circuit television
- Security
- Door access control
- Infant abduction control

Medical equipment

- Imaging equipment and systems
- Telemetry and patient monitoring
- Patient room furnishings
- Equipment management columns (booms)
- Sterilization and decontamination equipment
- Laboratory equipment

Source: Adapted from information available on the Web sites of Parsons Healthcare (http://www.meta-usa.com) and ACS Healthcare Solutions (http://www.acshealthcaresolutions.com).

Appendix P

Criteria for Selection of Medical Equipment and Products

ECRI staff offer some pointers for the selection of major medical equipment and single-use products, both of which are large cost items in a hospital's budget.

Medical Equipment

Key criteria include:

- Efficacy and effectiveness
- Performance
- Safety
- Reliability
- Features
- Ease of use
- Cost-effectiveness
- Service
- Training
- Continued user support

Efficacy is the ability of a diagnostic or therapeutic modality to fulfill its intended clinical purpose under optimum conditions. *Effectiveness* is the ability of a modality to fulfill its intended clinical purpose under real-world conditions and in day-to-day practice.

Performance is the measure of the ability of equipment to fulfill its intended purpose in conformity with its technical specifications or a standard.

Safety is a systems concept, not simply a product attribute.

Reliability is the measure of consistent performance and safety without failure.

Features are standard functional characteristics that define a type of device plus unique characteristics that differentiate it from other brands and models of its general type and purpose.

Ease of use reflects human factors design (ergonomics), user-friendliness of software, clarity of instructions, and intuitive operation by user.

Cost-effectiveness refers to the measure of health benefits for a given cost. Cost per use is usually more significant than initial purchase price.

Effective *service* has four components: documentation, parts, competent and responsive personnel, and factory support. Equipment service options include:

- Manufacturer or distributor
- Independent third-party service organization (ISO)
- In-house biomedical engineering technician(s)
- Regional biomedical technical center operated by the country's ministry of health or other governmental body

Training has two main objectives: to enable clinical users to apply the device safely and effectively to patients to achieve clinical objectives, and to enable engineering personnel to inspect, maintain, and service the device.

In addition to training, *continued user support* includes provision of documentation, replacement parts, software upgrades, and technical guidance to support continuing safe and effective device operation, as well as service and maintenance of the equipment.

Single-Use Products

Hospitals spend far more money for single-use products than for equipment each year. Some single-use products have a high unit cost (for example, pacemakers, cardiac catheters, and hip replacement components). Most single-use products have a low unit cost but are used in great quantities (for example, syringes, sutures, and needles).

Both equipment and single-use products can be lifesaving or present risks. Both are associated with design and manufacturing defects and user error.

Interactions between equipment and related single-use products (for example, dialyzers and infusion pumps) are sometimes the source of injury or death.

Criteria in the selection of single-use products include quality and price. Poor or inconsistent quality of some products, even though they may have the lowest unit cost, may actually increase the cost of serving patients (for example, scalp vein sets and IV catheters). There are great variations in prices paid for single-use products, even for neighboring hospitals purchasing similar quantities.

The key factors to minimize costs for single-use products are:

- Knowing what alternative suppliers charge for comparable products
- Knowing what other hospitals pay for the same products you are using
- Using strong bargaining skills based on having this up-to-date information
- Accessing this information from a consistent, reliable source (for example, PriceGuide)

Source: Adapted from ECRI, "Healthcare Technology: Equipment Procurement" (PowerPoint presentation, 2002).

Appendix Q

Sample Table for Construction Cost Estimates by Category

The following table shows the level of detail at which preliminary estimates for construction costs should be prepared. The items listed are provided for general information only and will need to be modified to meet the specific needs of each project.

No.	Construction Cost Estimates by Category Project: [ ] Hospital	Amount	%
1	**Piling and ground works**		
1.1	Excavation and filling		
1.2	Termite treatment		
1.3	Driven piling		
1.4	Timber piling		
1.5	Designed temporary works		
2	**Paving and roads**		
2.1	Roads and parking areas		
2.2	Pedestrian pavements		
2.3	Concrete kerbs and gate slabs		
2.4	Slab to loading bay area		
2.5	Storm drainage		
2.6	Manholes, covers, and gratings		
3	**Concrete work**		
3.1	Lean mix concrete		
3.2	Structural concrete grade [ ]		
3.3	Steel reinforcement to structure, grade [ ]		

No.	Construction Cost Estimates by Category Project: [ ] Hospital	Amount	%
3.4	Formwork for concrete		
3.5	Finishes to concrete slabs		
3.6	Vapor barrier below slab		
4	**Structural steelwork**		
4.1	Steel structures		
5	**Masonry**		
5.1	[ ] mm thick concrete blockwork walls		
5.2	[ ] mm clay brickwork to internal walls		
5.3	[ ] mm clay brickwork		
5.4	Builderswork in connection with M&E works		
6	**Woodwork**		
6.1	Dado protection rails		
7	**Roofing and waterproofing**		
7.1	Fluid-applied waterproofing (Sikaproof or similar)		
7.2	Xypex-type cement waterproofing		
7.3	External wall waterproofing system		
7.4	Roof accessories and drainage outlets		
7.5	Steel sheet roof and purlins to technical room		
7.6	Tent fabric		
8	**Partitions**		
8.1	Partition framing and lead lining		
8.2	Plasterboard partition linings		
9	**Thermal and acoustic insulation**		
9.1	Thermal insulation		
9.2	Acoustic insulation		
10	**Windows**		
10.1	Powder-coated aluminum external windows (opening)		
10.2	Internal windows (timber)		
11	**Glazing**		
11.1	[ ] mm tempered glass wall		
11.2	Glazing to external windows, [ ] mm laminated glass		
11.3	Glazing to internal windows, [ ] mm laminated glass		
11.4	Lead glass to X-ray areas		
11.5	Mirrors		
11.6	Glass balustrades		
12	**Doors**		
12.1	Doors, frames, and architraves		
12.2	Door hardware		

No.	Construction Cost Estimates by Category Project: [ ] Hospital	Amount	%
13	**Ceilings**		
13.1	Plasterboard ceilings		
13.2	Calcium silicate board ceilings		
13.3	Suspended tile ceilings, [ ] x [ ] mm		
14	**Plastering**		
14.1	[ ] mm cement render		
15	**Metalwork**		
15.1	Handrails, balustrades, and skirtings		
15.2	Galvanized steel		
15.3	Fencing and gates		
15.4	Fixing ceiling pendants		
15.5	Screens		
16	**Carpentry and fixed furniture**		
16.1	General cabinets (melamine-faced MDF, granite tops)		
16.2	Reception counters/fitments		
16.3	Vanity units and wash hand basins combined		
16.4	Toilet/shower partitions		
16.5	Curtain boxes and cill plates to windows		
16.6	Signage allowances		
16.7	Bathroom grab rails and accessories		
16.8	General equipment		
16.9	Bedroom furniture		
16.10	Blinds		
17	**Tiling and hard floor finishes**		
17.1	Ceramic wall tiling, [ ] x [ ] mm		
17.2	Ceramic NS homogeneous floor tiling, [ ] x [ ] mm		
17.3	Clinker tiles to roof terraces		
17.4	[ ] mm sealed granite finish to floors		
17.5	Accessories, matwells, stair treads		
17.6	Allowance for lift finishes		
18	**Flexible floor finishes**		
18.1	Carpet and underlay		
18.2	Antistatic conductive vinyl		
18.3	Vinyl flooring		
19	**Painting**		
19.1	Interior emulsion paint		
19.2	Exterior textured paint system (paint finish:)		
19.3	Painting to woodwork		

	Construction Cost Estimates by Category Project: [ ] Hospital		
No.		*Amount*	*%*
19.4	Painting to steelwork		
19.5	Road marking		
20	**Landscaping**		
20.1	Landscaping		
21	**Ancillary structures**		
21.1	Nuclear medicine and eye clinic (excluding services and piles)		
21.2	Gas, genset, transformer, and high-voltage switch building		
21.3	Entrance canopies		
21.4	Car and bike parking structures		
21.5	Garden area		
21.6	Guard house		
22	**Contingency: main contract**		
22.1	Contingency sum for buildingworks (at schematic design stage)		
23	**Preliminaries: main contract**		
23.1	Allowance for preliminaries		
24	**Subtotal: main contract**		

25	**Air conditioning and mechnical ventilation systems**		
25.1	Chiller plant system		
25.2	Air handling units		
25.3	Fan coil units		
25.4	Mechanical ventilation		
25.5	Building management system		
25.6	Miscellaneous		
26	**Plumbing and drainage**		
26.1	Sanitaryware and fittings		
26.2	Hot water system		
26.3	Water supply, pipes, and valves		
26.4	Drainage		
26.5	Water and wastewater treatment		
26.6	Miscellaneous		
27	**Fire protection**		
27.1	Hydrant and hose reels system		
27.2	Sprinkler system		
27.3	Miscellaneous		
28	**Electrical services**		
28.1	High-voltage connection, high-voltage switchboard, and transformer		

No.	Construction Cost Estimates by Category Project: [ ] Hospital	Amount	%
28.2	Standby generator		
28.3	Uninterruptible power system		
28.4	Distribution boards		
28.5	Light fittings (cf. switches)		
28.6	Power outlets		
28.7	Cables and conduits		
28.8	Earthing and lightning protection		
28.9	Telephone system		
28.10	Fire alarm system		
28.11	MATV/satellite TV system		
28.12	Public address		
28.13	Intercom		
28.14	Nurse call system		
28.15	Closed-circuit camera security system (CCTV)		
29	**Lift installation**		
29.1	Lift installation		
30	**Medical gases and vacuum systems**		
30.1	Medical gas systems		
31	**Allowance for nuclear medicine building**		
31.1	Contingency for nuclear medicine building		
32	**Provisions for mechanical and engineering works**		
32.1	Contingency sum for buildingworks (at schematic design stage)		
33	**Preliminaries: mechanical and engineering contract**		
33.1	Allowance for preliminaries		
34	**Subtotal: mechanical and engineering contract**		

35	**Grand total for construction (excluding VAT)**		**100**

Appendix R
International Competitive Bidding

When the World Bank provides financing to one of its member countries for investment projects, each project is governed by a legal agreement between the World Bank and the government agency that receives the funds. One of the key obligations in the loan agreement is that the country's government abide by the Bank's procurement policies. These are set forth in two documents: *Guidelines: Procurement under International Bank for Reconstruction and Development (IBRD) Loans* and *International Development Association (IDA) Credits* and *Guidelines: Selection and Employment of Consultants by World Bank Borrowers*.

One of the main responsibilities of the Bank's procurement sector is to help borrower countries improve their procurement systems. Sound public procurement policies and practices are essential to good governance. The purpose of the guidelines is to inform those carrying out a project that is financed in whole or in part by an IBRD loan or IDA credit of the arrangements to be made for procuring the goods and works, including related services, required for the project. The procurement guidelines include a description of international competitive bidding.

International competitive bidding is a process governing procurement in World Bank–financed projects and selection of consultants for the Bank's operational work. The objective is to provide all eligible prospective bidders with timely and adequate notification of a borrower's requirements and an equal opportunity to bid for the required goods and works. Details on international competitive bidding may be found on the World Bank Web site at http://web.worldbank.org/WBSITE/EXTERNAL/PROJECTS/PROCUREMENT/0,,contentMDK:20060844~menuPK:93305~pagePK:84269~piPK:84286~theSitePK:84266,00.html.

Although international competitive bidding and World Bank procurement processes are designed for and targeted to the public sector, the principles underlying them can be helpful in structuring procurement processes for private health care facilities. Ensuring broad market competition will tend to drive costs down and increase the quality of the products and services purchased.

Appendix S

Parsons META Hospital and Health Care Construction Pitfalls

Even with relatively detailed planning, construction projects in general, and hospital construction in particular, can get into difficulties. Parsons META offers the following examples of events or incidents that can cause delays and complications in construction. Some of the items have been discussed in chapters 7 and 9, but the list offered by Parsons META is presented here in its entirety for easy reference:

- Poor initial strategic planning assumptions (even though your operations may be growing very rapidly)
- Inadequate analysis of the current facility/site
- No real facility master plan done
- Alternatives never investigated (for example, another site or renovation versus new, and so forth)
- Unsubstantiated or nonexistent space program (hence a facility that is over-built)
- No one really in charge of the project (who has time and the right expertise)
- The wrong person or firm assumes control of the project
- Gaps in expertise (oops, did someone forget the geologic survey?)
- Poor-quality work by consultants
- Inadequate or poorly coordinated contract documents
- Lack of knowledge about the current codes and regulations impacting the facility
- Infighting among the key parties involved
- Inappropriate "cost segregation" resulting in inappropriate depreciation and excessive taxes

- Renting rather than buying equipment when renting does not make financial sense
- Exposure to litigation (quite common)
- Too many expensive change orders
- Duplicate fees
- Excessive fees (per consulting group)
- Cost overruns that cannot be financed

Careful and comprehensive planning and well-coordinated execution of the plans are the best way to ensure the successful completion of a hospital's construction!

Appendix T

Sample Job Description for Director of Nursing

The following job description for a director of nursing in a psychiatric hospital is used by the U.S. state of Connecticut. It is presented here as a general example of how a job description for professional hospital staff might be structured.

Purpose of Class

In the Department of Mental Health, Connecticut Valley Hospital, Norwich Hospital and Fairfield Hills Hospital, this class is accountable for directing nursing services.

Supervision Received

Receives administrative or executive direction from the Superintendent or other administrator of higher grade; receives functional supervision from the Chief and Assistant Chief of Mental Health Nursing Services.

Supervision Exercised

Directs managerial, professional, and other staff in the Department of Nursing.

Examples of Duties

Directs the staff and operation of the nursing department; coordinates, plans, and manages nursing department activities; formulates program goals and objectives; makes staff assignments; develops or assists in the development of related policy; interprets and administers pertinent laws; evaluates staff; prepares or assists in the preparation of the department budget; maintains contacts with individuals both within and outside of the department who might impact on program activities; participates in the recruitment and retention programs; protects human and civil rights of both patients/clients and staff; recommends disciplinary action; reviews and submits all periodic nursing reports; may represent the facility in meetings of professional or community organizations; may be appointed to standing committees; may participate in research activities; performs related duties as required.

Minimum Qualifications Required

Knowledge, skills, and ability: Considerable knowledge of principles and practices of psychiatric nursing; considerable knowledge of nursing administration; knowledge of and ability to apply management principles and techniques; knowledge of interviewing techniques; knowledge of current developments in field of nursing; knowledge of research procedures as applied to nursing; considerable interpersonal skills; considerable written and oral communication skills.

Experience and training: Three (3) years' experience in psychiatric hospital nursing in a managerial capacity at or above the level of Director of Nursing 1 (Psychiatric).

Special Requirement

1. Incumbents in this class must possess and retain a license as a registered professional nurse in Connecticut.
2. Incumbents in this class may be required to travel.

Source: State of Connecticut, Department of Administrative Services, http://www.das.state.ct.us/HR/jobspec/JobDetail.asp?FCC=1637.

Appendix U

10 Rules for Planning a Hospital

Joel J. Nobel, MD

The following list of 10 "dos and don'ts" is intended to help the first-time entrepreneur approach a hospital project realistically.

Don't:

- Forget that hospitals are very complex and challenging to plan, construct, equip, staff, and operate.
- Forget that construction and equipping a new hospital is only 4 percent of the lifetime cost of the facility, and planning is only a tiny percentage of that 4 percent.
- Try to save money up front by skimping on planning, especially on the feasibility study and project brief. Doing so will prove self-defeating and more costly in the end.
- Employ an architectural or engineering firm unless it has substantial recent experience in designing hospitals and the experienced staff is still available.
- Allow one powerful physician to dominate the planning process and distort the long-term priorities of the facility.

Do:

- Involve knowledgeable physicians, nurses, hospital administrators, and facility and biomedical engineers in the planning process.

- Be sure, at each planning stage, that you understand the financial tradeoffs between one-time project costs and long-term recurring operating costs. Saving money up front may cost far more later.
- Budget 10–15 percent of total anticipated project cost for unexpected contingencies.
- Remember that just as in medical care itself, effective planning requires a wide range of specialist consultants. Typical specialists required to design and construct a hospital properly include acoustic, biomedical, communications, electrical, mechanical, site, structural and waste management engineers; medical planners and medical equipment planners; hospital architects; and project managers, among others.
- Employ an independent medical equipment planner. Do not expect equipment suppliers to act in your best interest by offering a "free" planning service.

Suggested Reading

Agarwal, Amar. "Eight Steps Towards Building a World Class Facility." *Express Healthcare Management (Mumbai)*, August 31. http://www. expresshealthcaremgmt.com/20020831/hospinfra6.shtml. Reprinted in *Financial Risk Management*, ed. R. Bhaskaran (Hyderabad, India: ICFAI University Press, 2004).

American Institute of Architects. *Guidelines for Design and Construction of Health Care Facilities*. New York: American Institute of Architects and Facilities Guidelines Institute, 2006.

Assefzadeh, Saeed. "Assessing the Need to Establish New Hospitals." *Eastern Mediterranean Health Journal* 2, no. 2 (1996): 334–39. http://www.emro. who.int/publications/emhj/0202/23.htm.

Becker, Gregory C., and Bruce Ente. *Licensing and Accreditation Manual for Hospitals*. Prepared for USAID by Abt Associates, JCAHO, and the Committee for Accreditation and Licensing, Kyrgyz Republic, 1995. http://www.health-mgt.com/tech_papers/Hospital%20Accreditation%2 0Manual.pdf.

Capital Management Branch, Department of Human Services. *Capital Development Guidelines*. Melbourne: State Government of Victoria, Australia, 2005. http://www.dhs.vic.gov.au/pdfs/capdev/.

Dunlop, David W., and J. M. Martins, eds. *An International Assessment of Health Care Financing: Lessons for Developing Countries*. EDI Seminar Series. Washington, DC: World Bank, 1995.

Gapenski, Louis C. *Financial Analysis and Decision Making for Healthcare Organizations: A Guide for the Healthcare Professional*. Chicago: Healthcare Financial Management Association and Irwin Professional Publishing, 1997.

Griffin, Charles C. "Strengthening Health Services in Developing Countries through the Private Sector." Discussion Paper 4, International Finance Corporation, Washington, DC, 1989.

Harding, April, and A. S. Preker, eds. *Private Participation in Health Services.* Washington, DC: World Bank, 2003.

Kleczkowski, B. M., and R. Pibouleau, eds. *Approaches to Planning and Design of Health Care Facilities in Developing Areas.* 5 vols. Geneva: World Health Organization, 1976.

Lemle, J. Stuart. "Creating Successful Healthcare Delivery Facilities in Emerging Markets." *International Health Care Business Strategies Newsletter* 2 (3) (2001). http://www.rubcap.com/creating.html.

Lethbridge, Jane. "Forces and Reactions in Healthcare: A Report on Worldwide Trends for the PSI Health Services Taskforce." Public Services International Research Unit, School of Mathematical Sciences, University of Greenwich, London, 2002.

Marek, Tonia, C. O'Farrell, C. Yamamoto, and I. Zable. "Trends and Opportunities in Public-Private Partnerships to Improve Health Service Delivery in Africa." Africa Region Human Development Working Paper 93, World Bank, Washington, DC, 2005. http://siteresources.worldbank .org/INTAFRICA/Resources/wp93_health_service.pdf.

Marek, Tonia, C. Yamamoto, and J. Ruster. "Private Health: Policy and Regulatory Options for Private Participation." Public Policy for the Private Sector Note 264, World Bank, Washington, DC, 2003. http://rru .worldbank.org/Documents/PublicPolicyJournal/264Marek-063003.pdf.

Mills, Anne, and J. Broomberg. "Experiences of Contracting: An Overview of the Literature." WHO Macroeconomic, Health and Development Series Technical Paper 33, World Health Organization, Geneva, 1998.

Newbrander, William, ed. *Private Health Sector Growth in Asia: Issues and Implications.* Chichester, UK: John Wiley and Sons, 1996.

Preker, Alexander S., and A. Harding, eds. *Innovations in Health Service Delivery: The Corporatization of Public Hospitals.* Washington, DC: World Bank, 2003.

Prüss, Annette, E. Giroult, and P. Rushbrook, eds. *Safe Management of Wastes from Health-Care Activities.* Geneva: World Health Organization, 1999. http://www.healthcarewaste.org/en/documents.html?id=1.

Rea, John, Jeffrey J. Frommelt, and Malcolm D. MacCoun. *Building a Hospital: A Primer for Administrators.* Chicago: American Hospital Association, 1978.

Roa, Donna V., and A. Rooney. "Improving Health Services Delivery with Accreditation, Licensure, and Certification." *QA Brief* 8, no. 2 (Fall 1999). Quality Assurance Project, Bethesda, MD. http://www.qaproject .org/pubs/pdfs/engv8n2x.pdf.

Rohde, Deborah J., L. D. Prybil, and W. O. Hochkammer. *Planning and Managing Major Construction Projects: A Guide for Hospitals.* Ann Arbor, MI: Health Administration Press Perspectives, 1985.

Royer, Paul S. *Project Risk Management: A Proactive Approach.* Vienna, VA: Management Concepts, 2002.

Rushbrook, Philip, C. Chandra, and S. Gayton. *Starting Health Care Waste Management in Medical Institutions: A Practical Approach.* Health Care Waste Practical Information Series 1. Copenhagen: WHO Regional Office for Europe, 2000.

Savedoff, William, and Sekhri Neelam. "Private Health Insurance: Implications for Developing Countries." Discussion Paper 3-2004, World Health Organization, Geneva, 2004.

Scheckler, William E., D. Brimhall, A. Buck, B. Farr, C. Friedman, R. A. Garibaldi, P. A. Gross, J. Harris, W. J. Hierholzer, W. J. Martone, L. L. McDonald, and S. L. Solomon. "Requirements for Infrastructure and Essential Activities of Infection Control and Epidemiology in Hospitals: A Consensus Panel Report." *Infection Control and Epidemiogy* 19 (1998): 114–24; *American Journal of Infection Control* 26, no. 1 (1998): 47–60.

Schieber, George J., ed. *Innovations in Health Care Financing: Proceedings of a World Bank Conference, March 10–11, 1997.* World Bank Discussion Paper 365. Washington, DC: World Bank, 1997.

Useful Web Sites

- American Hospital Association. http://www.aha.org
- American Institute of Architects. http://www.aia.org
- Association for Professionals in Infection Control and Epidemiology. http://www.apic.org/AM/Template.cfm?Section=Home
- Association of American Physicians and Surgeons. http://www.aapsonline.org/
- Australian Healthcare Association. http://www.aushealthcare.com.au/
- Australian Private Hospitals Association. http://www.apha.org.au/
- C-Risk: Consultants in Risk Management. http://c-risk.com
- Capital Management Branch, Department of Human Services, State Government of Victoria, Australia. http://www.dhs.vic.gov.au/pdfs/
- ECRI Institute. http://www.ecri.org
- FindLaw for Business. http://smallbusiness.findlaw.com/starting-business/
- Global Health Resources. http://www.globalhealthresources.com
- Healthcare and Workforce Improvement Quality Assurance Project (USAID). http://www.qaproject.org/

- Healthcare Waste Management (WHO). http://www.healthcarewaste.org/en/115_overview.html
- Joint Commission International. http://www.jointcommissioninternational.org/
- Nous Hospital Consultants (P) Ltd. http://business.vsnl.com/nousdoc/hosp_org.html.
- Parsons META. http://www.meta-usa.com/index.html
- Public Services International Research Unit, University of Greenwich. http://www.psiru.org
- U.S. Small Business Administration. http://www.sba.gov
- UK Department for International Development (DFID) Health Resource Centre. http://www.dfidhealthrc.org/
- USAID Health Systems. http://www.usaid.gov/our_work/global_health/hs/index.html
- World Health Organization. http://www.who.int/
- WHO Regional Office for Africa. http://www.afro.who.int/
- WHO Regional Office for Americas. http://www.paho.int/
- WHO Regional Office for Europe. http://www.euro.who.int/
- WHO Regional Office for the Eastern Mediterranean. http://www.emro.who.int/
- WHO Regional Office for South-East Asia. http://www.searo.who.int/
- WHO Regional Office for the Western Pacific. http://www.wpro.who.int/